EMPOWERED OR LEFT BEHIND

Focused on the United States, this book summarizes the secondary impacts of COVID-19 due to the increased use of technology. Establishing the global response of social distancing, mandates for non-essential business, and working from home, the book centers on the disparate guidance provided domestically at the state and local levels. Marginalized populations are highlighted to identify areas where technology facilitated access and reach or contributed to difficulties catapulted by digital literacy or digital access issues. To explain how people may have been empowered or left behind due to new and unique reliance on technology, this book is structured based on the social determinants of health domains. Specifically, this book explains how technology was an umbrella domain that impacted every aspect of life during the pandemic, including access, use, adoption, and digital literacy, and digital equity, as well as privacy and security concerns. Given this book's focus on the impacts to marginalized populations, there is a thread throughout the book related to the use of technology to perpetuate hate, discrimination, racism, and xenophobic behaviors that emerged as a twin pandemic during COVID-19. Part I explains the defining differences between primary and secondary impacts, as well as the unique guidelines adopted in each state. Part II of the book is focused on specific domains, where each chapter is dedicated to topics including economic stability through employment, education, healthcare, and the social/community context through access to services. Part III focuses on unique technological considerations related to COVID-19, such as mobile health-related apps and privacy or security issues that may have posed barriers to the adoption and use of technology. Finally, the book ends with a conclusion chapter, which explicitly explains the advantages and disadvantages of technology adoption during COVID-19. These exposed benefits and challenges will have implications for policies, disaster management practices, and interdisciplinary research.

EMPOWERED OR LEFT BEHIND

Use of Technology During COVID-19

DeeDee M. Bennett Gayle
Xiaojun (Jenny) Yuan

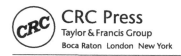

CRC Press
Taylor & Francis Group
Boca Raton London New York

CRC Press is an imprint of the
Taylor & Francis Group, an **informa** business

Designed cover image: Shutterstock Images

First edition published 2024
by CRC Press
2385 Executive Center Drive, Suite 320, Boca Raton, FL 33431

and by CRC Press
4 Park Square, Milton Park, Abingdon, Oxon, OX14 4RN

CRC Press is an imprint of Taylor & Francis Group, LLC

© 2024 DeeDee M. Bennett Gayle and Xiaojun (Jenny) Yuan

Library of Congress Cataloging-in-Publication Data
Names: Gayle, DeeDee Bennett, author. | Yuan, Xiaojun (Jenny), author.
Title: Empowered or left behind : use of technology during COVID-19 /
DeeDee Bennett Gayle, Xiaojun (Jenny) Yuan.
Description: First edition. | Boca Raton : CRC Press, 2023. | Includes
bibliographical references and index.
Identifiers: LCCN 2022062073 (print) | LCCN 2022062074 (ebook) | ISBN
9781032334981 (hardback) | ISBN 9781032335001 (paperback) | ISBN
9781003319894 (ebook)
Subjects: LCSH: COVID-19 Pandemic, 2020---Influence. | COVID-19 Pandemic,
2020---Social aspects. | Computer literacy--Social aspects.
Classification: LCC RA644.C67 G395 2023 (print) | LCC RA644.C67 (ebook) |
DDC 362.1962/4144--dc23/eng/20230420
LC record available at https://lccn.loc.gov/2022062073
LC ebook record available at https://lccn.loc.gov/2022062074

ISBN: 978-1-032-33498-1 (hbk)
ISBN: 978-1-032-33500-1 (pbk)
ISBN: 978-1-003-31989-4 (ebk)

DOI: 10.1201/9781003319894

Typeset in Caslon
by SPi Technologies India Pvt Ltd (Straive)

Contents

Acknowledgment

The premise of this work started in 2020 during the height of the COVID-19 pandemic and amid the many changes undertaken to minimize the spread of the virus. We secured a workgroup award to examine the technological innovations during COVID-19 from the Natural Hazards Center in Colorado as part of the larger National Science Foundation's CONVERGE initiative. Following this workgroup award, the authors received modest COVID-related grants from SUNY (State University of New York) and the University at Albany, SUNY President's Initiative on Minority Health Disparities Seed funding. The support of these awards allowed us to see the impact of technology during COVID more broadly. This also challenged us to consider the implications for reverting to our pre-COVID normal and deliberate about technology use post-COVID. Since we both study vulnerable populations, we wanted to expose how they are empowered or not in their use of technology during the lengthiest disaster in our lifetime. We are thankful for the support that each of the research awards provided us. We also received assistance from several research assistants and want to thank Natasha Edwards, Yvonne Dadson, Sean Li, Erin Li, and Austin Grattan.

Finally, without our families' love, support, and encouragement this manuscript would not have come to fruition. Special thank you to our spouses, Richard Gayle and Ming Li, and our children (some of whom served as research assistants), Sean Li, Erin Li, and Kingston Gayle. And a special thank you to Marie Bennett for her support and to our extended families.

About the Authors

DeeDee M. Bennett Gayle is Associate Professor and Director of the Extreme Events, Social Equity, and Technology (E²SET) Lab in the College of Emergency Preparedness, Homeland Security, and Cybersecurity at the University at Albany, State University of New York. Her interdisciplinary research focuses on the individual and household disaster impacts for vulnerable populations and how technologies may be leveraged to increase resilience. She has secured research grants and contracts, including from the National Science Foundation, Federal Emergency Management Agency, and the Department of Homeland Security. With over 50 publications, her work is published in various journals, and she has presented at several conferences related to communications, disasters, disability, diversity, wireless technology, and future studies. She is co-editor of an edited book volume on information behavior. Dr. Bennett Gayle received her PhD from Oklahoma State University in Fire and Emergency Management. She has a unique academic background having received both her MS in Public Policy and BS in Electrical Engineering from the Georgia Institute of Technology.

Xiaojun (Jenny) Yuan is an Associate Professor in the College of Emergency Preparedness, Homeland Security, and Cybersecurity at the University at Albany, State University of New York. Her research interests include both Human Computer Interaction and Information Retrieval, with the focus on user interface design and evaluation and human information behavior. Dr. Yuan has secured research grants and contracts from the Institute of Museum and Library Services, Department of Education in New York State and University at Albany. She published extensively in journals in information retrieval and human computer interaction, and conferences in computer science and information science, and is co-editor of the edited book volume *Social Vulnerability to COVID-19: Impacts of Technology Adoption and Information Behavior* with Springer Nature Publishing. She serves an Editorial Board member of *Aslib Journal of Information Management* (AJIM) and *Annual Review of Information Science and Technology* (ARIST), and a Board member of the International Chinese Association of Human Computer Interaction. Dr. Yuan received her PhD from Rutgers University at the School of Communication and Information and PhD from the Chinese Academy of Sciences in the Institute of Computing Technology. She received her MS in Statistics from Rutgers University and ME and BE in Computer Application from Xi'an University of Science & Technology in China.

PART I
GOVERNMENT RESPONSE AND IMPACTS

1

INTRODUCTION

Primary and Secondary Effects of COVID-19

"This pandemic has magnified every existing inequality in our society – like systemic racism, gender inequality, and poverty."

Melinda Gates (2020)

Beginning in late 2019, the virus SARS-CoV2 spread throughout the world and caused respiratory distress similar to the flu but with a significantly higher mortality rate. The virus was commonly known as COVID-19. This virus strain initially seemed to have the most damaging effects on older adults and individuals with preexisting conditions. Across the world, over six million people have died after contracting this disease as of 2022 (CSSE at JHU, 2022). Nearly 465 million cases of infection were reported in the first two years. In March of 2022, the global rate of new cases averaged nearly two million every 24 hours. Within the United States (U.S.), there were nearly one million deaths and 79 million cases (as of March 2022), making it the country with the most cases and deaths in the world (Connor, 2020). However, the rates of infection and mortality were not a steady, continuous climb; instead, there were ebbs and flows (or periods when infections skyrocketed and other times when infection rates were low). The protracted length of the pandemic and the waves of heightened alert about increasing infection provided ample time for people to become lax in their use of personal protective gear, such as masks. It was not uncommon in the U.S. to see mask mandates implemented and then removed, only to be implemented again. Initially, older adults and those with preexisting conditions were thought to be most at risk of infection; however, as the virus spread, it became more evident that racial and ethnic minorities were also at higher risk. These populations collectively comprised over a third of the U.S. population in 2019 and were more prone to be infected by this virus, with more

DOI: 10.1201/9781003319894-2

Table 1.1 Estimated Number and Percentage of Older Adults (65 Years or Older) and Racial Minorities under 65 Years Old in the U.S. (2019)

DEMOGRAPHICS[a]	TOTAL US POPULATION (2019)[a] = 328,239,523			
	RAW ESTIMATE TOTAL	RAW ESTIMATE (>65)	RAW ESTIMATE (<65)	% TOTAL POPULATION
Older Adults in the U.S. (>65 years)	54,074,028	54,074,028	–	16.5%
African American or Black (<65 years)	41,989,671	–	38,798,456	11.8%
Asian American (<65 years)	18,636,984	–	17,127,388	5.2%
Native American and Alaskan Native (<65 years)	2,847,336	–	2,528,711	0.8%
Native Hawaiian or Pacific Islander (<65 years)	628,683	–	569,123	0.2%
Hispanic or Latino (<65 years)[b]	*60,481,746*	–	*55,842,913*	*17.0%*
Total	–	54,074,028	59,023,678	34.5%

[a] *Source:* U.S. Census Bureau, 2019 American Community Survey 1-Year Estimates, https://data.census.gov/cedsci/table?q=United%20States&t=-01&tid=ACSSPP1Y2019.S0201
[b] The Hispanic or Latino population is not counted in the total here, given that Hispanic/Latino ethnicity can be selected across multiple races.

severe impacts, including a higher mortality rate. As shown in Table 1.1, by calculating the number of older adults (individuals over 65 years old) and racial minorities (under 65 years old) equates to 34.5% of the total U.S. population (without including Hispanic or Latino ethnic groups in the calculation, in which one can also be a member one or more racial categories). Throughout the pandemic, the media focus has been predominantly on the primary effects of COVID-19. However, even early on (during the spring of 2020), disaster researchers were very much aware that there would also be secondary impacts that would likely disproportionately affect marginalized populations (which include racial and ethnic minorities and older adults).[1]

Marginalization occurs when there are groups of people who have less access to resources, power, or opportunities. Typically, access is limited through discriminatory practices, prejudicial procedures, systems of racist policies, or individual biases. In the U.S., these groups often include racial and ethnic minorities, people with disabilities, low-income populations, children, as well as older adults (Bennett, 2010; Fothergill et al., 1999; Thomas et al., 2009; Wisner et al., 2004). Through the lens of the COVID-19 pandemic, discriminatory practices, procedures, policies, and biases impacted the lives of several populations, thus increasing the risk of infection for so many. Well-documented accounts from research have underscored this increased risk (Devakumar et al., 2020; Ransing et al., 2020; Ruiz et al., 2020). These risks were due to both primary and secondary impacts from COVID-19.

1.1 Primary and Secondary Impacts of COVID-19

Disparities during disasters are often segmented into primary and secondary impacts, with primary impacts indicating casualties, deaths, or damage directly due to the hazard in question. For COVID, the primary impacts were infection, hospitalization, or death due to the virus (Clay & Rogus, 2021). In contrast, secondary impacts have typically indicated concerns related to the social determinants of health, such as food insecurity, employment, living conditions, education, and access to specific services (Clay & Rogus, 2021). During COVID, both the primary and secondary impacts of the virus and the U.S. response were exposed as particularly difficult for marginalized populations. There were more reported deaths and infections in areas with higher proportions of African American populations (Millett et al., 2020). Increased exposure to the virus for essential workers also tends to be from ethnic minority or low-income populations (Reid et al., 2021). For example, COVID-19 mortality was higher among non-Hispanic or Latino (NH) African Americans compared with NH White Americans given the high correlation between essential worker employment among African Americans (Rogers et al., 2020). Hispanic and Latino Americans were also at greater risk of infection for similar reasons (Cheng et al., 2020; Gonzalez et al., 2021; Trick et al., 2021). At least one study questioned whether Hispanic populations were at greater risk of differential outcomes after COVID infection, noting the higher rates of ICU admissions (Nanchal et al., 2022). Among Native Americans, the primary impacts were more dire, with those living on reservation lands at increased risk of infection (Leggat-Barr et al., 2021; Yellow Horse et al., 2022). Some of the related factors to account for the disparities included increased co-morbidities, lower socioeconomic status, and the inability to social distance (Chang et al., 2021; Cheng et al., 2020; Gonzalez et al., 2021; Leggat-Barr et al., 2021; Millett et al., 2020; Qeadan et al., 2021; Trick et al., 2021).

Beyond contracting the virus, however, there were many more secondary impacts that had lasting effects on marginalized populations, some correlated with the increased reliance on and use of broadband wireless technologies. Mental health suffered amid the pandemic among racial and ethnic minorities (Novacek et al., 2020), children (Imran et al., 2020), people with disabilities (Jesus et al., 2021), and older adults (Vahia et al., 2020). Lost wages, economic insecurity, and unemployment were also increased concerns for so many (Acs & Karpman, 2020; Blustein et al., 2020; Gezici & Ozay, 2020; Kong & Prinz, 2020), including racial and ethnic minorities (Gezici & Ozay, 2020), and older adults (Li & Mutchler, 2020). Tangentially, food insecurity and energy insecurity were major concerns, as well, especially among the same populations (Memmott et al., 2021; Morales et al., 2021).

Furthermore, interpersonal violence increased, such as physical fighting among groups of individuals (Mazza et al., 2020). Social distancing did not help to reduce family violence, domestic violence, interpersonal violence, or hate-based violence, which affected people with disabilities (Lund, 2020), women (Roesch et al., 2020), children (Cappa & Jijon, 2021), and ethnic minorities, predominately African American and Asian American populations (Gover et al., 2020).

1.2 Vulnerability Literature and Theories

The idea that certain populations may be more vulnerable during disasters or extreme events is not new. In fact, disaster literature has long discussed the potential for socially vulnerable populations to be disproportionately impacted (directly and indirectly) by a variety of hazards in preparation for, during the response to, and amid recovery of an incident (Bennett, 2010, 2020; Thomas et al., 2009; Wisner, 2016). Several theories, frameworks, and models have been proposed to explain the disparate impacts.

The *social vulnerability theory* posits that disaster-related social vulnerability is related to the people and their characteristics, situations, perceptions, or knowledge, which causes them to be at an increased risk prior to, during, and after a disaster (Fatemi et al., 2017; Thomas et al., 2009; Wisner, 2016; Wisner, Blaikie & Cannon, 2004). This vulnerability can be influenced by individual-level factors such as employment, education, finances, family structure, or living conditions. It can also be influenced by macro-level forces, such as population growth, investment in preparedness, government structures, or medical services.

The *socio–political–ecology theory* states that those who are marginalized before a disaster occurs (or under blue-sky conditions) are likely to have disproportionate difficulties during and after a disaster. The assumption is that the difficulties are due to a scarcity of resources, which creates competition for resources during the disaster, producing a segment of winners and losers. Quite often, the losers in this competition are marginalized populations.

The *Pressure and Release Model (PAR model)*, developed by Wisner et al. (2004), theorized that disaster risk could be explained as an equation; combining the hazard and vulnerability would increase one's risk (see Equation 1.1), where the risk (R) is due to vulnerability (V), and where the hazard (H) can be from natural or human-made incidents, covering all types of hazards, including pandemics, drought, wildfires, earthquakes, hurricanes, and terrorist attacks, among others. In this equation, exposure is captured within vulnerability. The progression of vulnerability is based on individual livelihoods or unsafe conditions, dynamic forces, and root causes (Wisner et al., 2004). The PAR model has elements of Bronfenbrenner's Ecological Systems Theory (Bronfenbrenner, 1979), which considers vulnerability impacts at the micro- (individual level), meso- (neighborhood, church), exo- (workplace, hospital), and macro-systems (policies, laws, and customs) level (Eriksson et al., 2018).

$$R_{Disaster} = H \times V \tag{1.1}$$

The *Lens of Vulnerability* was developed to discuss the most vulnerable time for housing recovery, but in doing so, it explains how a lack of access to certain resources before a disaster can exacerbate vulnerability during the recovery stage of a disaster (Peacock et al., 2014). The most vulnerable time is after impact and before recovery, in which the access to resources is quite low for all households affected by the disaster.

The *Sustainable Livelihoods Approach* (SLA) was initially developed to outline the factors affecting poverty and food insecurity (Haidar & Centre, 2009; Massoud et al., 2016). Within this model, several types of livelihood assets can work together to reduce vulnerability. The livelihoods include financial (includes wealth, savings, income, and/or credit), natural (connected to the land, soil, fisheries, and water), human (usually related to skills and health), social (often related to networks, connection, community, and trust), and physical (typically referred to as the assets connected to the built environment – transport, housing, sanitation). This approach has also been used to explore the adverse impacts of disasters (Cannon et al., 2003; Kelman & Mather, 2008; Sanderson, 2000).

Several more recent studies have focused on *social capital*, or the lack thereof; and its relation to risk (Chriest & Niles, 2018; Makridis & Wu, 2021; Nyahunda & Tirivangasi, 2021; Rivera & Nickels, 2014). Social capital comes in a variety of forms, including linking, bonding, bridging, cognitive and structural (Nakagawa & Shaw, 2004; Phillips, 2009). Bonding social capital is where people from similar cultures, workplaces, characteristics, and/or faith traditions come together to work to solve wicked problems such as disaster resilience. Bridging social capital includes multidisciplinary approaches, working across differences and finding similarities. Linking social capital involves creating collaboration between organizations, government, and community members. Cognitive social capital is about gaining new knowledge and learning about perspectives and attitudes within the community to promote recovery. Structural social capital is about understanding the roles and responsibilities of individuals in charge of community and/or recovery efforts. Studies that focus on social capital have noted that many of the most vulnerable rely on certain forms of social capital to access resources. Lack of these types of capital can further disadvantage certain communities.

Though these models and frameworks provide an explanation of the increased vulnerability among certain groups, they do not identify how technology or digital literacy may have an impact. However, several additional studies have focused on how different information and communications technologies (ICTs) may contribute to the disparate impacts (Bennett et al., 2017; Bennett & LaForce, 2019; Gjøsæter et al., 2018, 2019; LaForce et al., 2016; Radianti et al., 2017). In the public health literature, *Social Determinants of Health* (SDH) are often used to show how multiple dimensions of an individual's life can contribute to adverse health outcomes and often leads to disparate impacts after disasters. Similar to the SLA framework, the SDH crosses over

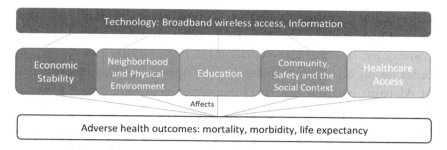

Figure 1.1 Proposed extended model of Social Determinants of Health (SDH). (Adopted from Benda et al. (2020), source from American Medical Association (Bennett et al., 2020.)

five (albeit slightly different) domains: financial, education, healthcare, neighborhood/built environment, and social/community. Additionally, much like the PAR model, these dimensions include individual-, meso-, and macro-level forces, from ecology theory. Interestingly, updated models of the ecology theory have included a techno-subsystem to emphasize the increasing importance and influence of technology (G. M. Johnson, 2010; Johnson & Puplampu, 2008). Again, SDH does not initially factor in the progression of technology or the increased reliance on technology for nearly every aspect of life, including across the five domains. However, arguments have discussed digital access or technology as a super SDH, crossing all five domains; see Figure 1.1 (Benda et al., 2020; Bennett et al., 2018; Clare, 2021; Early & Hernandez, 2021; Sieck et al., 2021).

1.3 Technology as a "Super" Social Determinant of Health

As a "super" social determinant of health (SDH), access to technology (digital access) impacts nearly all other social determinants; this was especially true amid COVID (Benda et al., 2020; Bennett et al., 2018; Clare, 2021; Early & Hernandez, 2021; Sieck et al., 2021). At the height of the pandemic, there were periods of "lock-down" in the U.S., which varied from state-to-state. During this lock-down period, state governors and local municipalities issued executive orders mandating people stay at home, and for nonessential businesses to close. For example, on March 19, 2020, the Governor of California issued an order for all individuals to stay at home; the next day, the

Governor of New York issued the "New York on PAUSE" executive order. On March 23, the Governor of Washington issued a stay-at-home order. By April 1, the Governor of Pennsylvania issued a similar order for all 67 counties. Likewise, on April 4, 2020, the Governor of Alabama issued a Stay-at-Home Order statewide. Some of these stay-at-home executive orders lasted over 200 days. These mandates forced most individuals to continue their daily activities (work, school, and recreation) all or in part online. Digital access and the use of technology became paramount during these varied orders. More information about the impacts of having varied state orders is discussed in Chapter 2. As much as the policy and cross-state variations impacted use and access of technology, preexisting digital divide and issues of achieving digital equity were concerns among marginalized populations (Dubois et al., 2021).

1.4 Digital Divide and Digital Equity

The conversation surrounding digital or device access did not originate during the pandemic. These discussions were ongoing long before and have focused on the digital divide to achieve some semblance of digital equity. The concept of the *Digital Divide* states that because of the increasing reliance of broadband wireless-based information and communication technologies (ICTs), those without access are disadvantaged (Cullen, 2001; van Dijk, 2006). Therefore, the divide occurs in the gap between those with access and those without. Ironically, individuals excluded or increasingly disadvantaged are often the same marginalized populations most at-risk during disasters. These populations include people with disabilities, racial and ethnic minorities, low-income, and older adults, among others. As Cullen (2001) noted, technology does not eliminate preexisting social inequities, and new technology does not always replace old technology. Therefore, the focus on leveraging new or better technologies may further disadvantage at-risk populations. *Digital Equity* is a call to action and a goal to achieve (Cox, 2008). For example, digital literacy must increase among the most disadvantaged groups to reduce the digital divide. Therefore, the digital equity goal (or call to action) is to increase access to information, services, and resources, which are increasingly accessible through broadband-wireless-based ICTs.

During the pandemic, access to several services required the use of technology. For some, the inability to use certain technologies caused secondary impacts such as the inability to find employment, access social services, connect with mental health professionals, or complete educational studies (Dubois et al., 2022; Yuan et al., 2022). For example, Gupta and Jawanda (2020) noted that the closure of schools eliminated the ways in which many children accessed the Internet. "Due to school closures, the learning gap will widen between children from low and high socioeconomic backgrounds" (Gupta & Jawanda, 2020, p1). More information about the impacts (on students, teachers, and parents) of having temporary remote instruction during COVID is discussed in Chapter 3. Children, however, were not the only individuals to have adverse impacts due to the increased use of technology over the pandemic. Migrant and rural populations (Chillag & Lee, 2020; Lee et al., n.d.) and people with disabilities (Armitage & Nellums, 2020; Bennett Gayle et al., 2021; Jesus et al., 2021; Lund et al., 2020) often had difficulties related to the digital divide and lack of digital inclusion. Some populations, however, found that the new and evolving ways in which technology was deployed during the pandemic was a unique benefit to them. Mobile health (and other variations of telehealth) reached much needed populations, e-commerce-based businesses saw a boom in activity, and telework opportunities opened possibilities for employment that were not readily accessible prior to COVID-19. Hence the title of this book. While some felt empowered by technology, others might have been left behind.

1.5 Overview of This Book

The goal of this book is to introduce readers to the types of secondary impacts of the COVID-19 pandemic, which were related to the near ubiquitous use of technology. Both the benefits and the barriers are highlighted throughout this book, identifying where the use of technology may have empowered individuals or communities, as well as where some populations were further disenfranchised. Throughout the book the pandemic is referred to in the past tense; however, at the time of this writing, the pandemic was still ongoing. As the authors commenced writing in March of 2022 there were 465 million cases worldwide, and by December of 2022 there were 645 million cases (CSSE at JHU, 2022). The death count in December of 2022 was over 6.6 million cases globally, with over 1 million from the U.S. alone (CSSE at JHU, 2022). This book is still timely, because though the pandemic was still ongoing, many of the policies and mandates restricting movement were relaxed in the U.S. These policies led most to embrace the use and implementation technologies across the SDH domains. While another publication may focus on the link between the mandates and individual impacts, this book only discusses the mandates to provide context for why so many different technologies were relied upon.

The organization of the book is segmented by areas of daily living (i.e., domains from the SDH), which were altered during the response and mitigation efforts. These efforts required populations to social distance (isolate and quarantine) and increased the use of broadband wireless–based software and devices. The book is structured so that readers can focus on one social domain or all, prioritizing the importance of different chapters. If readers are interested in how the use of technologies for education shifted amid the pandemic, they may want to focus solely on Chapter 5. Similarly, if interested in the impacts on employment and businesses, focus on Chapters 3 and 4. However, collectively, the book is written to provide an overview of how technology shifts amid the pandemic led to varying outcomes across the five SDH domains. The book is written for anyone interested in revisiting the impacts of the pandemic using the lens of technology use and adoption.

In this first chapter, the disparities in infection and mortality rates in the United States were introduced, along with additional challenges during the pandemic. The secondary impacts were also discussed to highlight their significance and disproportionate impact on some populations more than others. While this first chapter introduces the reader to the various impacts marginalized populations have had during the pandemic, the second chapter identifies how the impacts are related to disparate response efforts across state governments in the United States. In Chapter 2, additional challenges faced by individuals due to the difference in federal, state, and local mandates are discussed. The differing mandates led to geographic disparate use and adoption across some domains. These first two chapters (related to government response and impacts) set the stage for the subsequent benefits and challenges discussed throughout the rest of the book in terms of education, employment, and access to social and governmental services during the pandemic.

Part II of the book focuses on each social determinant of health domain, in which the use of technology may have fundamentally changed livelihoods for some people. In Chapter 3, the impacts to economic stability are explored along with the unequal impact on women and minority led business. In this chapter, the impacts on individuals, households, and small businesses that may have previously relied on foot traffic are discussed. Chapter 4 focuses on the use of technology to work from home, especially for those not considered essential workers. Chapter 5 features the reliance on technology for the continuance of education in K-12 and post-secondary institutions. In Chapter 6, other daily activities, such as access to gyms, grocery, and stores, were impacted by the stay-at-home measures and how technology was used as a workaround. Also included in Chapter 6 are examples of different access to government and organizational services, as well as technology leveraged to influence community safety. In Chapter 7, the new adoptions of personal technological devices to access healthcare services are explored. Chapter 7 includes topics such as the access to new mobile applications for e-health to increase access to providers for non-acute cases.

Part III of the book discusses unique technological considerations due to COVID-19 and the path forward. As technological innovations increased during the pandemic, adoption and use of technology changed. In Chapter 8, readers will learn about the health-related technological innovations used specifically for COVID. Perhaps some of these innovations will be long-lasting, and if so, how widely will they be adopted? Quickly developed telehealth services, contact tracing applications, and digital certificates for vaccinations caused concerns for data privacy and information security. Chapter 9 provides an overview of the various privacy and security concerns that occurred at the individual level for populations using various devices across SDH domains. Finally, Chapter 10 provides a summary of the entire book, highlighting the significant advantages and disadvantages of the rapid, ubiquitous use of technology to solve the social distancing and social isolation necessities amid the pandemic. By the end of this book, the reader should be able to identify populations who were empowered and populations who were left behind in certain aspects of their lives as technological reliance increased to reduce the spread of COVID-19.

Note

1 COVID-19 Working Groups for Public Health and Social Science Research https://converge.colorado.edu/resources/covid-19/working-groups/

References

Acs, G., & Karpman, M. (2020). Employment, income, and unemployment insurance during the COVID-19 Pandemic: Findings from the May 14–27 Coronavirus tracking survey. *Urban Institute*, 1–11. https://www.urban.org/sites/default/files/publication/102485/employment-income-and-unemployment-insurance-during-the-covid-19-pandemic.pdf

Armitage, R., & Nellums, L. B. (2020). The COVID-19 response must be disability inclusive. *The Lancet Public Health*, *5*(5), e257. https://doi.org/10.1016/S2468-2667(20)30076-1

Benda, N. C., Veinot, T. C., Sieck, C. J., & Ancker, J. S. (2020). Broadband internet access is a social determinant of health! *American Journal of Public Health*, *110*(8), 1123–1125. https://doi.org/10.2105/AJPH.2020.305784

Bennett, D. (2010). State emergency plans: Assessing the inclusiveness of vulnerable populations. *International Journal of Emergency Management*, *7*(1), 100.

Bennett, D. (2020). Five years later: Assessing the implementation of the four priorities of the Sendai framework for inclusion of people with disabilities. *International Journal of Disaster Risk Science*, *11*(2), 155–166.

Bennett, D., & LaForce, S. (2019). Text-to-action: Understanding the interaction between accessibility of Wireless Emergency Alerts and behavioral response. In *Risk communication and community resilience* (pp. 9–26). Routledge.

Bennett, D., Phillips, B. D., & Davis, E. (2017). The future of accessibility in disaster conditions: How wireless technologies will transform the life cycle of emergency management. *Futures*, *87*, 122–132.

Bennett Gayle, D., Yuan, X., & Knight, T. (2021). The coronavirus pandemic: Accessible technology for education, employment, and livelihoods. *Assistive Technology*, 1–8. https://doi.org/10.1080/10400435.2021.1980836

Bennett, N., Brown, M., Green, T., Hall, L., & Winkler, A. (2018). Addressing social determinants of health (SDOH): Beyond the clinic walls. Retrieved from American Medical Association: https://edhub.ama-assn.org/stepsforward/module/2702762

Blustein, D. L., Duffy, R., Ferreira, J. A., Cohen-Scali, V., Cinamon, R. G., & Allan, B. A. (2020). Unemployment in the time of COVID-19: A research agenda. *Journal of Vocational Behavior, 119*, 103436. https://doi.org/10.1016/j.jvb.2020.103436

Bronfenbrenner, U. (1979). *The ecology of human development: Experiments by nature and design.* Harvard University Press.

Cannon, T., Twigg, J., & Rowell, J. (2003). Social vulnerability, sustainable livelihoods and disasters. *Report to DFID Conflict and Humanitarian Assistance Department (CHAD) and Sustainable Livelihoods Support Office, 93*, 1–63.

Cappa, C., & Jijon, I. (2021). COVID-19 and violence against children: A review of early studies. *Child Abuse & Neglect, 116*, 105053. https://doi.org/10.1016/j.chiabu.2021.105053

Chang, T. S., Ding, Y., Freund, M. K., Johnson, R., Schwarz, T., Yabu, J. M., Hazlett, C., Chiang, J. N., Wulf, D. A., Antonio, A. L., Ariannejad, M., Badillo, A. M., Balliu, B., Berkovich, Y., Broudy, M., Dang, T., Denny, C., Eskin, E., Halperin, E., … Pasaniuc, B. (2021). Pre-existing conditions in Hispanics/Latinxs that are COVID-19 risk factors. *iScience, 24*(3), 102188. https://doi.org/10.1016/j.isci.2021.102188

Cheng, K. J. G., Sun, Y., & Monnat, S. M. (2020). COVID-19 death rates are higher in rural counties with larger shares of blacks and hispanics. *The Journal of Rural Health, 36*(4), 602–608. https://doi.org/10.1111/jrh.12511

Chillag, K. L., & Lee, L. M. (2020). Synergistic disparities and public health mitigation of COVID-19 in the rural United States. *Journal of Bioethical Inquiry, 17*(4), 649–656. https://doi.org/10.1007/s11673-020-10049-0

Chriest, A., & Niles, M. (2018). The role of community social capital for food security following an extreme weather event. *Journal of Rural Studies, 64*, 80–90. https://doi.org/10.1016/j.jrurstud.2018.09.019

Clare, C. A. (2021). Telehealth and the digital divide as a social determinant of health during the COVID-19 pandemic. *Network Modeling Analysis in Health Informatics and Bioinformatics, 10*(1), 26. https://doi.org/10.1007/s13721-021-00300-y

Clay, L. A., & Rogus, S. (2021). Primary and secondary health impacts of COVID-19 among minority individuals in New York State. *International Journal of Environmental Research and Public Health, 18*(2), Article 2. https://doi.org/10.3390/ijerph18020683

Connor, R. (2020, April 8). *Coronavirus: Timeline of the global spread of COVID-19 – DW – 04/08/2020.* Dw.Com. https://www.dw.com/en/coronavirus-timeline-of-the-global-spread-of-covid-19/g-52145412

Cox, M. (2008). *Researching IT in Education* (Vol. 20, pp. 965–981). https://doi.org/10.1007/978-0-387-73315-9_61

CSSE at JHU. (2022). *COVID-19 Map* [Map]. Johns Hopkins University. https://coronavirus.jhu.edu/map.html

Cullen, R. (2001). Addressing the digital divide. *Online Information Review, 25*(5), 311–320. https://doi.org/10.1108/14684520110410517

Devakumar, D., Shannon, G., Bhopal, S. S., & Abubakar, I. (2020). Racism and discrimination in COVID-19 responses. *The Lancet, 395*(10231), 1194.

Dubois, E., Bright, D., & Laforce, S. (2021). Educating minoritized students in the United States during COVID-19: How technology can be both the problem and the solution. *IT Professional, 23*(2), 12–18. https://doi.org/10.1109/MITP.2021.3062765

Dubois, E., Yuan, X., Bennett, D., Khurana, P., Knight, T., Laforce, S., Turetsky, D., & Wild, D. (2022). Socially vulnerable populations adoption of technology to address lifestyle changes amid COVID-19 in the US. *Data and Information Management, 100001.* https://doi.org/10.1016/j.dim.2022.100001

Early, J., & Hernandez, A. (2021). Digital disenfranchisement and COVID-19: Broadband internet access as a social determinant of health. *Health Promotion Practice, 22*(5), 605–610. https://doi.org/10.1177/15248399211014490

Eriksson, M., Ghazinour, M., & Hammarström, A. (2018). Different uses of Bronfenbrenner's ecological theory in public mental health research: What is their value for guiding public mental health policy and practice? *Social Theory & Health, 16*(4), 414–433. https://doi.org/10.1057/s41285-018-0065-6

Fatemi, F., Ardalan, A., Aguirre, B., Mansouri, N., & Mohammadfam, I. (2017). Social vulnerability indicators in disasters: Findings from a systematic review. *International Journal of Disaster Risk Reduction, 22*, 219–227.

Fothergill, A., Maestas, E. G., & Darlington, J. D. (1999). Race, ethnicity and disasters in the United States: A review of the literature. *Disasters, 23*(2), 156–173.

Gezici, A., & Ozay, O. (2020). *How race and gender shape COVID-19 unemployment probability.* https://doi.org/10.2139/ssrn.3675022

Gjøsæter, T., Radianti, J., & Chen, W. (2018). Universal design of ICT for emergency management: A systematic literature review and research agenda. In *Universal Access in Human-Computer Interaction. Methods, Technologies, and Users: 12th International Conference, UAHCI 2018, Held as Part of HCI International 2018, , Las Vegas, NV, USA, July 15-20, 2018, Proceedings, Part I 12* (pp. 63–74). Springer International Publishing. https://uia.brage.unit.no/uia-xmlui/bitstream/handle/11250/2596600/UD-v10-CR-final.pdf?isAllowed=y&sequence=2

Gjøsæter, T., Radianti, J., & Chen, W. (2019). *Understanding situational disabilities and situational awareness in disasters*, Proceedings of the 16th ISCRAM Conference – València, Spain May 2019, https://idl.iscram.org/files/terjegjosaeter/2019/1924_TerjeGjosaeter_etal2019.pdf

Gonzalez, C. J., Aristega Almeida, B., Corpuz, G. S., Mora, H. A., Aladesuru, O., Shapiro, M. F., & Sterling, M. R. (2021). Challenges with social distancing during the COVID-19 pandemic among Hispanics in New York City: A qualitative study. *BMC Public Health, 21*(1), 1946. https://doi.org/10.1186/s12889-021-11939-7

Gover, A. R., Harper, S. B., & Langton, L. (2020). Anti-Asian hate crime during the COVID-19 pandemic: Exploring the reproduction of inequality. *American Journal of Criminal Justice, 45*(4), 647–667. https://doi.org/10.1007/s12103-020-09545-1

Gupta, S., & Jawanda, M. (2020). The impacts of COVID-19 on children. *Acta Paediatrica, 109.* https://doi.org/10.1111/apa.15484

Haidar, M., & Centre, U. D. D. (2009). *Sustainable livelihood approaches* : https://digitallibrary.un.org/record/679330

Imran, N., Zeshan, M., & Pervaiz, Z. (2020). Mental health considerations for children & adolescents in COVID-19 Pandemic. *Pakistan Journal of Medical Sciences*, *36*(COVID19-S4), S67–S72. https://doi.org/10.12669/pjms.36.COVID19-S4.2759

Jesus, T. S., Bhattacharjya, S., Papadimitriou, C., Bogdanova, Y., Bentley, J., Arango-Lasprilla, J. C., Kamalakannan, S., & The Refugee Empowerment Task Force, I. N. G. of the A. C. of R. M. (2021). Lockdown-related disparities experienced by people with disabilities during the first wave of the COVID-19 pandemic: Scoping review with thematic analysis. *International Journal of Environmental Research and Public Health*, *18*(12), Article 12. https://doi.org/10.3390/ijerph18126178

Johnson, G. M. (2010). Internet use and child development: The techno-microsystem. *Australian Journal of Educational and Developmental Psychology*, *10*, 32–43.

Johnson, G. M., & Puplampu, K. P. (2008). Internet use during childhood and the ecological techno-subsystem. *Canadian Journal of Learning and Technology*, *34*(1). https://eric.ed.gov/?id=EJ1073829

Kelman, I., & Mather, T. A. (2008). Living with volcanoes: The sustainable livelihoods approach for volcano-related opportunities. *Journal of Volcanology and Geothermal Research*, *172*(3–4), 189–198.

Kong, E., & Prinz, D. (2020). Disentangling policy effects using proxy data: Which shutdown policies affected unemployment during the COVID-19 pandemic? *Journal of Public Economics*, *189*, 104257. https://doi.org/10.1016/j.jpubeco.2020.104257

LaForce, S., Bennett, D. M., Linden, M., Touzet, C., & Mitchell, H. (2016). *Optimizing accessibility of wireless emergency alerts: 2015 survey findings.*

Lee, J. G. L., LePrevost, C. E., Harwell, E. L., Bloss, J. E., Cofie, L. E., Wiggins, M. F., & Firnhaber, G. C. (n.d.). Coronavirus pandemic highlights critical gaps in rural Internet access for migrant and seasonal farm-workers: A call for partnership with medical libraries. *Journal of the Medical Library Association: JMLA*, *108*(4), 651–655. https://doi.org/10.5195/jmla.2020.1045

Leggat-Barr, K., Uchikoshi, F., & Goldman, N. (2021). COVID-19 risk factors and mortality among Native Americans. *Demographic Research*, *45*, 1185–1218.

Li, Y., & Mutchler, J. E. (2020). Older adults and the economic impact of the COVID-19 pandemic. *Journal of Aging & Social Policy*, *32*(4–5), 477–487. https://doi.org/10.1080/08959420.2020.1773191

Lund, E. M. (2020). Interpersonal violence against people with disabilities: Additional concerns and considerations in the COVID-19 pandemic. *Rehabilitation Psychology*, *65*(3), 199–205. https://doi.org/10.1037/rep0000347

Lund, E. M., Forber-Pratt, A. J., Wilson, C., & Mona, L. R. (2020). The COVID-19 pandemic, stress, and trauma in the disability community:

A call to action. *Rehabilitation Psychology, 65*(4), 313–322. https://doi.org/10.1037/rep0000368

Makridis, C. A., & Wu, C. (2021). How social capital helps communities weather the COVID-19 pandemic. *PLoS One, 16*(1), 1–18.

Massoud, M. A., Issa, S., Fadel, M. E., & Jamali, I. (2016). Sustainable livelihood approach towards enhanced management of rural resources. *International Journal of Sustainable Society, 8*(1), 54. https://doi.org/10.1504/IJSSOC.2016.074947

Mazza, M., Marano, G., Lai, C., Janiri, L., & Sani, G. (2020). Danger in danger: Interpersonal violence during COVID-19 quarantine. *Psychiatry Research, 289*, 113046. https://doi.org/10.1016/j.psychres.2020.113046

Memmott, T., Carley, S., Graff, M., & Konisky, D. M. (2021). Sociodemographic disparities in energy insecurity among low-income households before and during the COVID-19 pandemic. *Nature Energy, 6*(2), Article 2. https://doi.org/10.1038/s41560-020-00763-9

Millett, G. A., Jones, A. T., Benkeser, D., Baral, S., Mercer, L., Beyrer, C., Honermann, B., Lankiewicz, E., Mena, L., Crowley, J. S., Sherwood, J., & Sullivan, P. S. (2020). Assessing differential impacts of COVID-19 on black communities. *Annals of Epidemiology, 47*, 37–44. https://doi.org/10.1016/j.annepidem.2020.05.003

Morales, D. X., Morales, S. A., & Beltran, T. F. (2021). Racial/ethnic disparities in household food insecurity during the COVID-19 pandemic: A nationally representative study. *Journal of Racial and Ethnic Health Disparities, 8*(5), 1300–1314. https://doi.org/10.1007/s40615-020-00892-7

Nakagawa, Y., & Shaw, R. (2004). Social capital: A missing link to disaster recovery. *International Journal of Mass Emergencies and Disasters, 22*.

Nanchal, R., Patel, D., Guddati, A. K., Sakhuja, A., Meersman, M., Dalton, D., & Kumar, G. (2022). Outcomes of Covid 19 patients—Are Hispanics at greater risk? *Journal of Medical Virology, 94*(3), 945–950. https://doi.org/10.1002/jmv.27384

Novacek, D. M., Hampton-Anderson, J. N., Ebor, M. T., Loeb, T. B., & Wyatt, G. E. (2020). Mental health ramifications of the COVID-19 pandemic for black Americans: Clinical and research recommendations. *Psychological Trauma : Theory, Research, Practice and Policy, 12*(5), 449–451. https://doi.org/10.1037/tra0000796

Nyahunda, L., & Tirivangasi, H. M. (2021). Harnessing of social capital as a determinant for climate change adaptation in Mazungunye communal lands in Bikita, Zimbabwe. *Scientifica, 1–9*. https://doi.org/10.1155/2021/8416410

Peacock, W. G., Van Zandt, S., Zhang, Y., & Highfield, W. E. (2014). Inequities in long-term housing recovery after disasters. *Journal of the American Planning Association, 80*(4), 356–371.

Phillips, B. D. (2009). *Disaster recovery*. Auerbach Publications.

Qeadan, F., VanSant-Webb, E., Tingey, B., Rogers, T. N., Brooks, E., Mensah, N. A., Winkfield, K. M., Saeed, A. I., English, K., & Rogers, C. R. (2021). Racial disparities in COVID-19 outcomes exist despite comparable Elixhauser comorbidity indices between Blacks, Hispanics, Native

Americans, and Whites. *Scientific Reports*, *11*(1), Article 1. https://doi. org/10.1038/s41598-021-88308-2

Radianti, J., Gjøsæter, T., & Chen, W. (2017). Universal design of information sharing tools for disaster risk reduction. *International Conference on Information Technology in Disaster Risk Reduction*, 81–95.

Ransing, R., Ramalho, R., de Filippis, R., Ojeahere, M. I., Karaliuniene, R., Orsolini, L., da Costa, M. P., Ullah, I., Grandinetti, P., & Bytyçi, D. G. (2020). Infectious disease outbreak related stigma and discrimination during the COVID-19 pandemic: Drivers, facilitators, manifestations, and outcomes across the world. *Brain, Behavior, and Immunity*, *89*, 555.

Reid, A., Ronda-Perez, E., & Schenker, M. B. (2021). Migrant workers, essential work, and COVID-19. *American Journal of Industrial Medicine*, *64*(2), 73–77. https://doi.org/10.1002/ajim.23209

Rivera, J. D., & Nickels, A. E. (2014). Social capital, community resilience, and faith-based organizations in disaster recovery: A case study of Mary Queen of Vietnam Catholic Church. *Risk, Hazards & Crisis in Public Policy*, *5*(2), 178–211.

Roesch, E., Amin, A., Gupta, J., & Garcia-Moreno, C. (2020). Violence against women during covid-19 pandemic restrictions. *BMJ*, *369*. https://doi. org/10.1136/bmj.m1712

Rogers, T. N., Rogers, C. R., VanSant-Webb, E., Gu, L. Y., Yan, B., & Qeadan, F. (2020). Racial disparities in COVID-19 mortality among essential workers in the United States. *World Medical & Health Policy*, *12*(3), 311–327. https://doi.org/10.1002/wmh3.358

Ruiz, N. G., Horowitz, J. M., & Tamir, C. (2020, July 1). Many black and Asian Americans say they have experienced discrimination amid the COVID-19 outbreak. *Pew Research Center's Social & Demographic Trends Project.* https://www.pewresearch.org/social-trends/2020/07/01/many-black-and-asian-americans-say-they-have-experienced-discrimination-amid-the-covid-19-outbreak/

Sanderson, D. (2000). Cities, disasters and livelihoods. *Risk Management*, *2*(4), 49–58.

Sieck, C. J., Sheon, A., Ancker, J. S., Castek, J., Callahan, B., & Siefer, A. (2021). Digital inclusion as a social determinant of health. *Npj Digital Medicine*, *4*(1), Article 1. https://doi.org/10.1038/s41746-021-00413-8

Thomas, D. S., Phillips, B. D., Fothergill, A., & Blinn-Pike, L. (2009). *Social vulnerability to disasters*. CRC Press.

Trick, W. E., Badri, S., Doshi, K., Zhang, H., Rezai, K., Hoffman, M. J., & Weinstein, R. A. (2021). Epidemiology of COVID-19 vs. influenza: Differential failure of COVID-19 mitigation among Hispanics, Cook County Health, Illinois. *PLoS One*, *16*(1), e0240202. https://doi. org/10.1371/journal.pone.0240202.

Vahia, I., Jeste, D., & Reynolds, C. (2020). Older adults and the mental health effects of COVID-19. *JAMA: Geriatrics*, *324*(22), 2253–2254. https://doi. org/10.1001/jama.2020.21753

van Dijk, J. A. G. M. (2006). Digital divide research, achievements and shortcomings. *Poetics*, *34*(4–5), 221–235. https://doi.org/10.1016/j.poetic. 2006.05.004

Wisner, B. (2016, August 31). *Vulnerability as concept, model, metric, and tool.* Oxford Research Encyclopedia of Natural Hazard Science. https://doi. org/10.1093/acrefore/9780199389407.013.25

Wisner, G. W., Blaikie, P., & Cannon, T. (2004). *At risk: Natural hazards, people's vulnerability and disasters.* Routledge.

Yellow Horse, A. J., Yang, T.-C., & Huyser, K. R. (2022). Structural inequalities established the architecture for COVID-19 pandemic among native Americans in Arizona: A geographically weighted regression perspective. *Journal of Racial and Ethnic Health Disparities, 9*(1), 165–175. https://doi. org/10.1007/s40615-020-00940-2

Yuan, X., Wu, D., & Bennett Gayle, D. (Eds.). (2022). *Social vulnerability to COVID-19: Impacts of technology adoption and information Behavior.* Springer.

2

COVID-19 US Response

"Be Safe, Be Smart, Be Kind."

Tedros Adhanom Ghebreyesus
WHO Director General (2020)

The federal response to the pandemic was slow. States had to react to the pandemic primarily on their own, which led to uneven public health response across the nation. As Haffajee and Mello (2020) mentioned, the shortcomings of the public health governance of US were exposed by COVID-19, and the federal, state, and local governments' powers divided because the virus was super transmissible and penetrated borders. In other words, the US response to COVID-19 was far from cohesive. The lack of inter-jurisdictional coordination between states made it challenging to successfully implement guidelines on social distancing and masking or adopt quarantine measures in places where the virus was quickly spreading. Despite that, by March 27, 2020, the federal government and all 50 states had declared emergencies for COVID-19. Within the emergency orders, guidelines included halting select commercial operations, limiting freedom of movement, reducing the size of gatherings, closing schools and non-essential businesses, or sheltering in place.

2.1 Public Health Guidance

There was a divergence of public health guidance at the state level. In December 2020, the World Health Organization (WHO) guidance stated that masks alone were not an effective measure to prevent uninfected people from catching the virus. Specifically, the December guidance stated that masks can protect others if the mask wearer is infected, protecting oneself from infection, or both (WHO, 2020). Per the guidance on the WHO website, masks act as a barrier to prevent the spread of the virus from the wearer to other individuals:

DOI: 10.1201/9781003319894-3

WHO advises that governments should encourage the use of non-medical fabric masks, which can act as a barrier to prevent the spread of the virus from the wearer to others where there are many cases of COVID-19, for people in the general public where physical distancing of at least 1 metre is not possible – such as, on public transport, in shops or in other confined or crowded environments.

(WHO, 2020)

Though masks could be used to protect oneself from catching the virus, early medical advice and risk communication messaging indicated that the mask was more likely to prevent the spread from an infected masked individual, rather than protect a masked person from catching the virus from an unmasked infected individual (Bryan Health, n.d.; *DHSS Insights*, 2020). In the US, many mask mandates were interpreted to mean those who were most at-risk should wear a mask, those infected, and everyone in healthcare settings. Amid the pandemic, various community mitigation policies were adopted by the states and localities, such as social distancing and face-masking (CDC, 2020; Hatef et al., 2021). However, the mitigation measures varied by geography in terms of content and timing. In some locations, masks were not mandated at the state level, only at the local level, such as Florida (JHU, 2022).

2.1.1 Social Distancing

Before therapeutics and the full capacity of contact tracing, COVID-19 mitigation strategies depended on social distancing policies to minimize the number of infected people and to reduce COVID-19-related morbidity and mortality (Ferguson et al., 2020). The timing, sequencing, and level of enforcement of social distancing policies varied in each state (Kaufman et al., 2021). The Centers for Disease Control and Prevention (CDC) offered guidance in response to COVID-19, but it was up to state and local governments to execute social distancing policies. Because of the nature of the SAR-CoV2 virus, the differences in states' implementation strategies led to disparity between states in the effectiveness of social distancing measures (Kaufman et al., 2021).

The direct impact of social distancing policies across states varied (see Figure 2.1), where "eleven states were estimated to have prevented

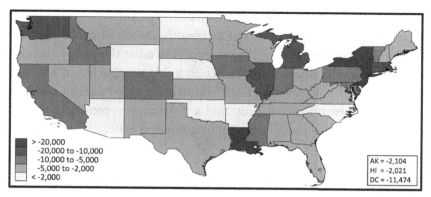

Notes: Figure generated using Stata 16.0 to present results of the authors' analysis of *New York Times* COVID-19 US database. Cumulative daily COVID-19 cases (January 21 to May 7, 2020) were estimated using a generalized linear model with a negative binomial distribution and a log link and offset to account for state population. For each state, we used the method of recycled predictions to compare predicted cumulative cases with social distancing compared to without social distancing at three weeks after the date of school closure. Estimates are presented in the supplemental material.

Figure 2.1   The impact of social distancing policies varied across states (Kaufman et al., 2021.)

more than 10,000 cases per 100,000 residents" (Kaufman et al., 2021, p. 5). While Figure 2.1 focuses on primary impacts, a host of secondary impacts also led to adverse health outcomes.

2.1.2 State Actions to Mitigate the Spread of COVID-19

Across the nation, not only did each state have different guidance; but in some states the delegation of guidance was at the local municipality level. This means that across jurisdictions in the same state and in neighboring states the guidance for COVID-19 varied (KFF, 2021). This contributed to a variety of disparate impacts based solely on geography, as there were over 89,004 local governments in the U.S. at the time (Census Bureau, 2012). The important decision to choose an appropriate time to end the community mitigation measures had very real consequences. The CDC initially suggested a 14-day downward trajectory of documented positive COVID-19 tests (percent of total) as the threshold to evaluate the best time to relax community mitigation measures (CDC, 2020, Hatef et al., 2021). However, some states did not follow the suggestion; instead, they moved forward with the relaxation of the measures without waiting for a consistent downward trend (Johns Hopkins University and Medicine, 2020; Boston University School of Public Health, 2020), discussed further in Box 2.1. The consequences were experienced at the individual and household levels, where the variance in guidance also led to a disparate use of technology across health domains (e.g., education, employment, and government services) and a difference in messaging based on geographic location all contributing to adverse health outcomes.

BOX 2.1   VARIED STATE GUIDANCE ON COVID-19

As of August 4, 2021, individuals were required to wear face masks in public locations (e.g., transportation, healthcare, schools, and other locations). But the guidance varied across states, and some cases were delegated locally. For example, some states pushed the decision-making guidance for COVID-19 to the local municipalities, such as Colorado and Nevada.

In New Mexico, some counties under turquoise-level restrictions allowed gatherings of up to 150 people. In Oregon, the restrictions on large indoor gatherings varied in terms of county risk level. In the 9 high-risk counties, gatherings were limited to 6 people; in the 5 moderate-risk counties, 8 people; and in the 22 lower-risk counties, 10 people. For travelers to Hawaii, if they register with the state and have a negative COVID-19 test before the departure, they may be able to stay away from the mandatory 14-day quarantine.

Source: KFF (2021). State Actions to Mitigate
the Spread of COVID-19

Research has proven the impact of implementation of mitigation policies had on decreasing COVID-19 prevalence, hospitalization, and death rates (Courtemanche et al., 2020; Xie et al., 2020; Badr et al., 2020; VoPham et al., 2020; Lyu and Wehby, 2020; Friedson et al., 2020). The negative impacts were indications of (1) the improper relaxation of the mitigation policies (Hatef et al., 2021); and (2) not following CDC guidelines (Kaufman et al., 2021). One mitigation effort ongoing throughout the pandemic was the dissemination of risk communication.

2.2 Messaging During COVID-19

During the pandemic, it was critical for the governments (at state and local levels) to decide how best to communicate appropriate messages with the public. Officials struggled with culturally competent messaging that effectively led to appropriate protective action, such as with the mask mandates (Ho & Huang, 2021; Martinelli et al., 2021). Previous research identified several factors related to cultural competency of risk messaging, such as cultural concerns of varying demographics (Crouse Quinn, 2008), culture (Kreuter & McClure, 2004), trust (Bennett Gayle & Yuan, 2022), and the disparities among different demographics (Brankston et al., 2021). Researchers also highlighted the challenges in expanding awareness and accessibility about public health and health-related social determinants (Niederdeppe et al., 2008). Furthermore, the protracted length of the pandemic (over 2 years) and seemingly seasonal changes with infections presented barriers with maintaining the attention and trust of the public, as guidance shifted in response (Sutton et al., 2020).

BOX 2.2   NEW YORK STATE ON PAUSE

(Policy That Assures Uniform Safety for Everyone)

Many cities and states were severely impacted by COVID-19. Among them was New York City (NYC), with a reported 164,505 cases, 42,417 hospitalizations, and 13,000 confirmed deaths as of April 30, 2020 (NYCDH, 2020), representing 16.4% of cases and 24.8% of deaths nationally (Lamb, Kandula, & Shaman, 2021). On March 22, 2020, former Governor Cuomo signed the "New York State on PAUSE" executive order, a ten-point policy to assure uniform safety for everyone. It included directives for non-essential businesses statewide to close in-office personnel functions effective at 8pm on Sunday, March 22. It also temporarily banned all non-essential gatherings of individuals of any size for any reason (NYS on Pause, 2020).

NYS on PAUSE was a method to mitigate the spread of the COVID-19 and is correlated to a significant decrease in travel time (Gao, Bernardes, Bian, Ozbay, & Iyer, 2020). The variance in travel time corresponded to governor's orders. In addition to NYS on PAUSE, former Governor Cuomo was readily featured on local and national broadcast news outlets daily to provide 111 briefings (between March 2 and June 19, 2020) with statistical measures of infections, hospital admissions, and mortality rates, as well as statewide mitigation measures, mandates, and changing guidance (Fink, 2020). Due to the reach of his briefings, many households in other states followed his advice.

Sutton (2021) pointed out that the protracted length of the pandemic would lead to message fatigue, where individuals choose not to heed advice due to the sheer influx of messaging on the topic. For example, in NY, former Governor Cuomo held over 100 daily press briefings during the height of the pandemic (Fink, 2020); see Box 2.2. By examining the relation between message fatigue and decision-making regarding the use of masks (Ball & Wozniak, 2021), social distancing (Seiter & Curran, 2021, Chou & Budenz, 2020), and vaccination (Chou & Budenz, 2020), researchers found that message fatigue and mistrust are barriers to appropriate decision-making regarding personal protective action during the pandemic. The adoption of these measures also differed among populations, and the differences can be attributed to health literacy and risk perception (Paakkari & Okan, 2020, Sutton et al., 2020, Benham et al., 2021).

2.3 Technology Used to Disseminate Messages

Several different technologies were used to disseminate COVID-19 messaging, such as television, mobile phone, social media, online media, radio, digital road signs, and mobile applications. Due to the unregulated user-generated content on social networks, mixed messages with information and misinformation occupied the internet (Garrett, 2020; Zarocostas, 2020; Xie et al., 2020). For instance, after having examined 1,000 randomly selected tweets about antibiotics,

Scanfeld, Scanfeld, and Larson (2010) reported that 700 of them (about 70%) contained medical misinformation or malpractice. Meanwhile, messaging and mandates were varied by location in the U.S., which in turn led to mixed messaging. The mixed messaging about mask usage, social distancing, and vaccination might also have caused mistrust (Ho & Huang, 2021, Shelus et al., 2020). For example, in November 2021 CDC issued guidance recommending vaccinations of all children 5 to 11; however, by March 2022, the Florida Department of Health stated that healthy children between 5 and 17 may not benefit from the COVID-19 vaccine (CDC, 2021; JHU, 2022).

Researchers recognized trust was a significant indicator of individual behavioral change (Zhao et al., 2020; Hughes & Chauhan, 2015; Liu et al., 2021). Yuan and White (2012) carried out user experiments to compare the health information behaviors of general users with medical professionals and found that trust is a key factor in users' selection of websites to search for health-related information. During COVID, Bennett Gayle and Yuan (2022) claimed that trust was related to the individual or organization disseminating the message, perception about risk and potential problems due to contracting the virus, or the efficacy of mitigating efforts, such as wearing a mask. Once available, the message dissemination measures expanded to include the use of a contact tracing app and digital vaccine passports (or certificates), as available by location (Benham et al., 2021). Again, the use of technology varied from state-to-state. With bill AL SB267, Alabama banned the use of vaccine passports in April 2021. Similar restrictions were issued in Arizona, Arkansas, Florida, Georgia, Idaho, Indiana, Iowa, North Dakota, South Carolina, South Dakota, and Texas (Davis, 2021).

2.3.1 *Health Literacy, Digital Literacy, and Trust*

Health literacy and personal risk perception were also important factors to individuals' decision-making about taking protective actions (Ironstone, 2022; Paakkari & Okan, 2020; Abrams & Greenhawt, 2020). Health literacy often changes from person to person and is correlated with demographic characteristics, including age (Sudore et al., 2006; Fleary & Ettienne, 2019), household income and education (Fleary & Ettienne, 2019), and certain racial and ethnic minorities (Van Servellen et al., 2003; Fleary & Ettienne, 2019). Similarly, risk perception varies among the population and is often correlated with certain demographic differences, as well (Olofsson & Rashid, 2011; Fleary & Ettienne, 2019).

At the very beginning of the pandemic, public health officials warned that specific populations were more at risk for infection to the virus. Much of the attention and public health messaging was focused on older adults, among other high-risk groups, and the messaging was primarily directed toward these populations (Shahid et al., 2020). In a survey study, Bennett Gayle and Yuan (2022) examined how older adults receive emergency communications disseminated about COVID-19. When asked about the most trusted individuals or organizations, by far, most of the respondents' trust messages sent through CDC (82%), State Governor Briefings (66%), and the World Health Organizations (65%); see Figure 2.2. For those who selected "other," responses ranged from employer, PubMed, *Science Magazine*, Stansberry Research reports, Dr. Fauci, Dr. Birx, specific shows on TV, and doctors interviewed on news shows. Scientists (or information from medical science) were not one of the primary trusted individuals as indicated by the respondents, though mentioned by some. Additionally, among those who selected State Governor Briefings, some participants outside of New York made a point to indicate that they specifically trusted the governor of New York.

Pearson's Chi-squared test results on the relationship between behavioral response with stakeholder perception showed significant

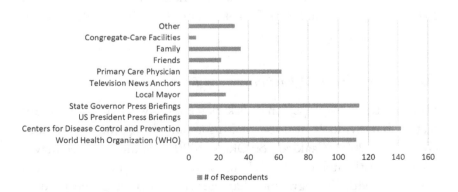

Figure 2.2 Trusted entities about the pandemic by number of respondents.

relationships between trust in WHO or the state governor and the decision to stay indoors, wear masks, and wear gloves. Additional relationships were found between trust in the CDC and the decision to stay indoors, and wear masks. Trust in the local mayor led to one significant behavioral change finding, which was to stay indoors. These findings emphasize the significant importance of the state and federal public health guidelines and individual decision-making.

2.3.2 Broadband Infrastructure

The necessity of broadband wireless technology expanded during the pandemic. While state guidance differed so did the way in which each state managed broadband deployment (Read & Gong, 2021). Additionally, the agencies responsible for the handling of the deployment varied with respect to goals, expectations, challenges, and potential investments. Table 2.1 shows how each state designed its broadband infrastructure. In this table, office is a consolidated sector for broadband projects, while an agency is a unit working on broadband projects (Read and Gong, 2021). Additionally, the task fund indicated an official team focused on broadband issues, while fund represented a resource to distribute grants across jurisdictions to provide broadband access to the public.

Several states did not establish centralized offices to manage broadband program, including Wyoming, Vermont, South Dakota, Rhode Island, Pennsylvania, Oklahoma, North Dakota, New Jersey, New Hampshire, Nevada, Nebraska, Montana, Mississippi, Iowa, Georgia, Delaware, Arizona, Alaska, and Alabama. Most of the states employed agencies to coordinate broadband program efforts, with the state of Mississippi as the only exception (Read and Gong, 2021).

2.4 Impacts of Guidance across the Health Domains

The variation of guidance did not only directly affect health outcomes, but they also affected social determinants of health domains. As noted in Chapter 1, the SDH domains indirectly lead to adverse health outcomes. These domains include education, employment, and daily activities.

Table 2.1   Four Primary Features of State Management
Broadband Deployment Available by State

STATE	OFFICE	AGENCY	TASK FORCE	FUND
Wyoming	No	Yes	Yes	Yes
Wisconsin	Yes	Yes	Yes	Yes
West Virginia	Yes	Yes	Yes	Yes
Washington	Yes	Yes	No	Yes
Virginia	Yes	Yes	Yes	Yes
Vermont	No	Yes	Yes	Yes
Utah	Yes	Yes	Yes	Yes
Texas	Yes	Yes	Yes	No
Tennessee	No	Yes	No	Yes
South Dakota	No	Yes	No	Yes
South Carolina	Yes	Yes	No	Yes
Rhode Island	No	Yes	No	No
Pennsylvania	No	Yes	No	Yes
Oregon	Yes	Yes	Yes	Yes
Oklahoma	No	Yes	Yes	Yes
Ohio	Yes	Yes	No	Yes
North Dakota	No	Yes	Yes	No
North Carolina	Yes	Yes	Yes	Yes
New York	Yes	Yes	No	Yes
New Mexico	Yes	Yes	Yes	Yes
New Jersey	No	Yes	Yes	No
New Hampshire	No	Yes	Yes	Yes
Nevada	No	Yes	Yes	Yes
Nebraska	No	Yes	Yes	Yes
Montana	No	Yes	Yes	Yes
Missouri	Yes	Yes	No	Yes
Mississippi	No	No	No	No
Minnesota	Yes	Yes	Yes	Yes
Michigan	Yes	Yes	Yes	Yes
Massachusetts	Yes	Yes	No	Yes
Maryland	Yes	Yes	Yes	Yes
Maine	Yes	Yes	No	Yes
Louisiana	Yes	Yes	Yes	Yes
Kentucky	Yes	Yes	Yes	Yes
Kansas	Yes	Yes	Yes	Yes
Iowa	No	Yes	Yes	Yes
Indiana	Yes	Yes	No	Yes
Illinois	Yes	Yes	Yes	Yes

(Continued)

Table 2.1 (Continued) Four Primary Features of State Management Broadband Deployment Available by

STATE	OFFICE	AGENCY	TASK FORCE	FUND
Idaho	Yes	Yes	Yes	Yes
Hawaii	Yes	Yes	Yes	Yes
Georgia	No	Yes	No	Yes
Florida	Yes	Yes	No	Yes
Delaware	No	Yes	Yes	Yes
Connecticut	Yes	Yes	No	No
Colorado	Yes	Yes	Yes	Yes
California	Yes	Yes	Yes	Yes
Arkansas	Yes	Yes	No	Yes
Arizona	No	Yes	No	Yes
Alaska	No	Yes	Yes	Yes
Alabama	No	Yes	Yes	Yes

(adapted from source: Read & Gong, 2021.)

2.4.1 Education

The pandemic changed the concept of education and the education system in the U.S. in various ways. All stakeholders, including teachers, administrators, students, and parents, were impacted by the federal and state guidance. Many of these changes contributed to one of the biggest educational crises in history (Karakose, 2021). In the U.S., after most of the stay-at-home orders in March 2020, nearly every school transformed to immediate remote instruction. Online meeting and teaching platforms (Zoom, Webex, Google Classrooms, Microsoft Teams, among others) dominated and reshaped the world of education.

The pandemic provided opportunities for education professionals to rethink how to redesign higher education and develop innovative teaching-learning strategies (Karakose, 2021). After having adapted to the fully online teaching and working format, some people realized the benefits and challenges of working from home while caring for children and family. For example, because of the pandemic, parents needed to spend more time at home, helping their children with schoolwork – which also impacted the labor market (Bacher-Hicks et al., 2020).

The secondary impacts from COVID on education were far-reaching (Karakose, 2021). In a study (Lee, Solomon, Stead, Kwon, & Ganti, 2021) on mental health of college students amid the COVID-19 pandemic, it was reported that the mental health status of college students has been most affected by their worries about the health of their loved ones, they are anxious about their continuing education remotely, lack of productivity at home, concerned about losing job and internship opportunities, and contracting the virus. Most importantly, many respondents indicated that their concern began when university campuses began to shut down. They also indicated concerns when states issued lockdown guidelines shortly after. These executive orders inevitably served as a turning point here.

2.4.2 Employment

Many technologies were leveraged to keep the business sector thriving, but again much of this occurred from homes. As governments implemented mandates for social distancing or segmenting industries into essential and non-essential statuses, broadband wireless technologies were adopted to comply. Contactless technologies were used to minimize employee exposure of essential workers, and digital monitoring technologies were used for employees working from home. However, many employees were laid off or furloughed during this time.

A global analysis of 20 democratic countries reported that 38 million (5.7%) of total workers applied for unemployment insurance due to the pandemic as of May 2020 (Rothwell, 2020). Whereas, there have been more than 40 million initial unemployment claims in the U.S. since mid-March 2020 (Reiniche, 2020). As can be seen from some labor-market data, the significant unemployment increases that are related to pandemic-related business closures in spring 2020 were mostly women and workers without four-year college degrees, as well as disproportionately racial and ethnic minority populations (Fairlie et al., 2020). Since low-income U.S. households commonly do not have much savings for emergent situations (Beshears et al., 2020), unemployment can cause financial distress and insecurity of food and housing (Bansak, & Starr, 2021).

2.4.3 Daily Activities

During COVID-19, recreational and fitness facilities pivoted to online avenues to continue offering their services. Places of worship streamed religious services through our phones, televisions, and computers. Some switched to free streaming-video services like PlutoTV and Tubi (Lachapelle, 2020), virtual worship or virtual fitness classes or mobile fitness apps to continue their daily exercise (Dubois et al., 2022). Since most recreational, fitness and religious activities were conducted online, some populations faced challenges of technology access and use, as well as the costs associated with such use (Dubois et al., 2022). The physical activity of many populations was reduced during the pandemic (Hoffman et al., 2021; The United Nations, 2020).

2.5 Summary

The U.S. COVID-19 response varied across states because of the constitutional nature of the government. This chapter discussed the guidelines on social distancing, and the state action to curb the spread of the virus. It addressed the importance for the governments (at state and local levels) to make decisions on public messaging and technologies that can be used to communicate appropriate and trustful messages to the public. More importantly, the variation of guidance impacted the social determinants of health domains, including education, employment, and daily activities. The connections between the social determinants of health will be discussed in more detail in subsequent chapters. The disparities for marginalized populations were exacerbated in each health domain. It is important to design and develop innovative tools that will allow employees, parents, students, and teachers to effectively pivot virtually, if needed. However, considering the digital divide and the negative impacts for certain populations. Therefore, it is critical for officials, policymakers, and educational administrators to adjust expectations.

References

Abrams, E. M., & Greenhawt, M. (2020). Risk communication during COVID-19. *The Journal of Allergy and Clinical Immunology: In Practice, 8*(6), 1791–1794.

Bacher-Hicks, A., Goodman, J., & Mulhern, C. (2020). Inequality in household adaptation to schooling shocks: covid-induced online learning engagement in real time. NBER Working paper, No. 27555.

Ball, H., & Wozniak, T. R. (2021). Why do some Americans resist COVID-19 prevention behavior? An analysis of issue importance, message fatigue, and reactance regarding COVID-19 messaging. *Health Communication*, *37*(14), 1812–1819.

Bansak, C., & Starr, M. (2021). Covid-19 shocks to education supply: how 200,000 US households dealt with the sudden shift to distance learning. *Review of Economics of the Household*, *19*(1), 63–90.

Benham, J. L., Lang, R., Kovacs Burns, K., MacKean, G., Léveillé, T., McCormack, B., ... & Marshall, D. A. (2021). Attitudes, current behaviours and barriers to public health measures that reduce COVID-19 transmission: A qualitative study to inform public health messaging. *PLoS One*, *16*(2), e0246941.

Bennett Gayle, D., & Yuan, X.-J. (2022). Older adults decision-making at the beginning of the COVID-19 pandemic. *The Journal of Human Ecological Assessment* (submitted).

Beshears, J., Choi, J., Iwry, J., John, D., Laibson, D., & Madrian, B. (2020). Building emergency savings through employer-sponsored rainy-day savings accounts. *Tax Policy and the Economy*, *34*(1), 43–90.

Boston University School of Public Health. 2020. COVID-19 US State Policy Database (CUSP) https://www.bu.edu/sph/2020/04/01/tracking-covid-19-policies/. Accessed on September 2, 2020.

Brankston, G., Merkley, E., Fisman, D. N., Tuite, A. R., Poljak, Z., Loewen, P. J., & Greer, A. L. (2021). Socio-demographic disparities in knowledge, practices, and ability to comply with COVID-19 public health measures in Canada. *Canadian Journal of Public Health*, *112*(3), 363–375.

Bryan Health. (n.d.). *Wearing a mask is not only important, it's life-saving*. Bryan Health. https://www.bryanhealth.com/coronavirus-clp/wearing-a-mask-is-not-only-important-its-life-saving/. Accessed on October 28, 2022.

Census Bureau. (2012). *Census bureau reports There are 89,004 local governments in the United States—Governments—Newsroom—U.S. Census Bureau*. US Census Bureau Public Information. https://www.census.gov/newsroom/releases/archives/governments/cb12-161.html

Centers for Disease Control and Prevention [CDC]. 2020. Severe outcomes among patients with coronavirus disease 2019 (COVID-19)—United States, February 12–March 16, 2020. https://www.cdc.gov/mmwr/volumes/69/wr/mm6912e2.htm. Accessed March 26, 2022.

Centers for Disease Control and Prevention [CDC] 2021. CDC recommends pediatric COVID-19 vaccine for children 5 to 11 years. https://www.cdc.gov/media/releases/2021/s1102-PediatricCOVID-19Vaccine.html Accessed November 21, 2022.

Crouse Quinn, S. (2008). Crisis and emergency risk communication in a pandemic: A model for building capacity and resilience of minority communities. *Health Promotion Practice*, *9*(4_suppl), 18S–25S.

Davis, Jr., E. (2021, June 1). These states have banned vaccine passports. https://www.usnews.com/news/best-states/articles/which-states-have-banned-vaccine-passports Accessed on November 21, 2022.

DHSS Insights: Wearing masks while playing sports and exercising strongly recommended. (2020, October 10). Alaska DHSS. https://content.govdelivery.com/accounts/AKDHSS/bulletins/2a5251e

Dubois, E., Yuan, X., Bennett, D., Khurana, P., Knight, T., Laforce, S., ... & Wild, D. (2022). Socially vulnerable populations adoption of technology to address lifestyle changes amid COVID-19 in the US. *Data and Information Management*, 6(2), *100001*.

Fairlie, R. W., Couch, K. A., & Huanan, X. (2020). The impacts of Covid-19 on minority unemployment: first evidence from April 2020 CPS microdata. NBER Working Paper No. w27246.

Ferguson, N. M., Laydon, D., Nedjati-Gilani, G., et al. (2020). Report 9: Impact of non-pharmaceutical interventions (NPIs) to reduce COVID-19 mortality and healthcare demand. Imperial College COVID-19 Response Team. https://spiral.imperial.ac.uk/handle/10044/1/77482

Fink, Z. (2020, June 18). *Cuomo Announces His Daily Coronavirus Briefings Will End.* https://www.ny1.com/nyc/all-boroughs/news/2020/06/18/cuomo-announces-his-daily-coronavirus-briefings-will-end-

Fleary, S. A., & Ettienne, R. (2019). Social disparities in health literacy in the United States. *HLRP: Health Literacy Research and Practice*, 3(1), e47–e52.

Gao, J., Bernardes, S. D., Bian, Z., Ozbay, K., & Iyer, S. (2020). Initial impacts of COVID-19 on transportation systems: A case study of the US epicenter, the New York metropolitan area. arXiv preprint arXiv: 2010.01168.

Garrett, L. (2020). COVID-19: The medium is the message. *Lancet*, *395*(10228), 942–943.

Haffajee & Mello (2020, May 28). Thinking globally, acting locally — The U.S. Response to Covid-19. *The New England Journal of Medicine*, *382*, e75. https://www.nejm.org/doi/full/10.1056/NEJMp2006740

Hatef, E., Kitchen, C., Chang, H. Y., Kharrazi, H., Tang, W., & Weiner, J. P. (2021). Early relaxation of community mitigation policies and risk of COVID-19 resurgence in the United States. *Preventive Medicine*, *145*, 106435.

Ho, A., & Huang, V. (2021). Unmasking the ethics of public health messaging in a pandemic. *Journal of Bioethical Inquiry*, *18*, 549–559.

Hoffman, G. J., Malani, P. N., Solway, E., Kirch, M., Singer, D. C., Kullgren, J. T. (2021). Changes in activity levels, physical functioning, and fall risk during the COVID-19 pandemic *Journal of the American Geriatrics Society*. https://doi.org/10.1111/jgs.17477

Hughes, A. L., & Chauhan, A. (2015). Online media as a means to affect public trust in emergency responders. In ISCRAM.

Ironstone, P. (2022). Critical communication studies and COVID-19: Mediation, discourse, and masks. In Elliott, C., Greenberg, J. (eds) *Communication and health* (pp. 315–333). Palgrave Macmillan, Singapore.

Johns Hopkins University and Medicine. JHU; Baltimore (MD). (2020). Coronavirus Resource Center. COVID-19 Dashboard by the Center for Systems Science and Engineering (CSSE) at Johns Hopkins University (JHU) https://coronavirus.jhu.edu/map.html Accessed on September 2, 2020.

Johns Hopkins University and Medicine. JHU; Baltimore (MD). (2022). Impact of Opening and Closing Decisions by state. COVID-19 Dashboard by the Center for Systems Science and Engineering (CSSE) at Johns Hopkins University (JHU) https://coronavirus.jhu.edu/data/state-timeline/new-confirmed-cases/florida/0. Accessed on November 21, 2022.

Karakose, T. (2021). The impact of the COVID-19 epidemic on higher education: Opportunities and implications for policy and practice. *Educational Process: International Journal, 10*(1), 7–12.

Kaufman, B. G., Whitaker, R., Mahendraratnam, N., Hurewitz, S., Yi, J., Smith, V. A., & McClellan, M. (2021). State variation in effects of state social distancing policies on COVID-19 cases. *BMC Public Health, 21*(1), 1–6.

KFF. (2021) State Actions to Mitigate the Spread of COVID-19 | KFF.

Kreuter, M. W., & McClure, S. M. (2004). The role of culture in health communication. *Annual Review of Public Health, 25*, 439–455.

Lachapelle, T. (2020). How covid-19 is changing entertainment, in five charts. Yahoo Finance (2020). https://finance.yahoo.com/news/covid-19-changing-entertainment-five-120029434.html

Lamb, M. R., Kandula, S., & Shaman, J. (2021). Differential COVID-19 case positivity in New York City neighborhoods: Socioeconomic factors and mobility. *Influenza and Other Respiratory Viruses, 15*(2), 209–217.

Lee, J., Solomon, M., Stead, T., Kwon, B., & Ganti, L. (2021). Impact of COVID-19 on the mental health of US college students. *BMC Psychology, 9*(1), 1–10.

Liu, Y., Qin, Z., Ye, Z., Zhang, X., & Meng, F. (2021). Explaining trust and consequences of COVID-19 rumors on social media: A SOR perspective.

Martinelli, L., Kopilaš, V., Vidmar, M., Heavin, C., Machado, H., Todorović, Z., … & Gajović, S. (2021). Face masks during the COVID-19 pandemic: a simple protection tool with many meanings. *Frontiers in Public Health*, 947. https://www.frontiersin.org/articles/10.3389/fpubh.2020.606635/full

Niederdeppe, J., Bu, Q. L., Borah, P., Kindig, D. A., & Robert, S. A. (2008). Message design strategies to raise public awareness of social determinants of health and population health disparities. *The Milbank Quarterly, 86*(3), 481–513.

NYCDH (2020). New York City Department of Health and Mental Hygiene. COVID 19 Data archive. https://www1.nyc.gov/site/doh/covid/covid-19-data-archive.page

NYS on Pause (2020). Governor Cuomo Signs the 'New York State on PAUSE' Executive Order | Governor Kathy Hochul (ny.gov)

Olofsson, A., & Rashid, S. (2011). The white (male) effect and risk perception: can equality make a difference? *Risk Analysis: An International Journal, 31*(6), 1016–1032.

Paakkari, L., & Okan, O. (2020). COVID-19: Health literacy is an underestimated problem. *The Lancet. Public Health*, *5*(5), e249.

Read, A., & Gong, L. (2021). Which States Have Dedicated Broadband Offices, Task Forces, Agencies, or Funds? A review of state strategies for improving access. Published on June 28, 2021 Updated: November 30, 2021 Which States Have Dedicated Broadband Offices, Task Forces, Agencies, or Funds? | The Pew Charitable Trusts (pewtrusts.org). Accessed on May, 31, 2022.

Rothwell, J. (2020, May 27). The effects of COVID-19 on international labor markets: An update. *Brookings.* https://www.brookings.edu/research/the-effects-of-covid-19-on-international-labor-markets-an-update/

Scanfeld, D., Scanfeld, V., & Larson, E. L. (2010). Dissemination of health information through social networks: Twitter and antibiotics. *American Journal of Infection Control*, *38*(3), 182–188.

Seiter, J. S., & Curran, T. (2021). Social-distancing fatigue during the COVID-19 pandemic: a mediation analysis of cognitive flexibility, fatigue, depression, and adherence to CDC guidelines. *Communication Research Reports*, *38*(1), 68–78.

Shahid, Z., Kalayanamitra, R., McClafferty, B., Kepko, D., Ramgobin, D., Patel, R., ... & Jain, R. (2020). COVID-19 and older adults: What we know. *Journal of the American Geriatrics Society*, *68*(5), 926–929.

Shelus, V. S., Frank, S. C., Lazard, A. J., Higgins, I. C., Pulido, M., Richter, A. P. C., ... & Hall, M. G. (2020). Motivations and barriers for the use of face coverings during the COVID-19 pandemic: Messaging insights from focus groups. *International Journal of Environmental Research and Public Health*, *17*(24), 9298.

Sudore, R. L., Mehta, K. M., Simonsick, E. M., Harris, T. B., Newman, A. B., Satterfield, S., ... & Health, Aging and Body Composition Study, (2006). Limited literacy in older people and disparities in health and healthcare access. *Journal of the American Geriatrics Society*, *54*(5), 770–776.

Sutton, J., Rivera, Y., Sell, T. K., Moran, M. B., Bennett Gayle, D. M., Schoch-Spana, M., Stern, E., & Turetsky, D. (2020). Longitudinal risk communication: A research agenda for communicating in a pandemic. *Health Security Journal.* https://www.liebertpub.com/doi/full/10.1089/hs.2020.0161

United Nations (2020). *The impact of COVID-19 on sport, physical activity and well-being and its effects on social development.* The United Nations. https://www.un.org/development/desa/dspd/2020/05/covid-19-sport/

Van Servellen, G., Brown, J. S., Lombardi, E., & Herrera, G. (2003). Health literacy in low-income Latino men and women receiving antiretroviral therapy in community-based treatment centers. *AIDS Patient Care and STDs*, *17*(6), 283–298.

World Health Organization. (2020). Rational use of personal protective equipment for coronavirus disease (COVID-19): Interim guidance, 27 February 2020 (No. WHO/2019- nCov/IPCPPE_use/2020.1). World Health Organization.

Xie, B., He, D., Mercer, T., Wang, Y., Wu, D., Fleischmann, K. R., … & Lee, M. K. (2020). Global health crises are also information crises: A call to action. *Journal of the Association for Information Science and Technology*, *71*(12), 1419–1423.

Yuan, X.-J., & White, R. (2012, May). Building the trail best traveled: Effects of domain knowledge on web search trailblazing. *Proceedings of the ACM SIGCHI Conference on Human Factors in Computing Systems (CHI 2012)*. Austin, Texas, USA.

Zarocostas, J. (2020). How to fight an infodemic. *Lancet*, *395*(10225), 676.

Zhao, E., Wu, Q., Crimmins, E. M., & Ailshire, J. A. (2020). Media trust and infection mitigating behaviours during the COVID-19 pandemic in the USA. *BMJ Global Health*, *5*(10), e003323.

PART II

TECHNOLOGY USE ACROSS THE HEALTH DOMAINS

3

BUSINESSES AND
SELF-EMPLOYMENT

"When we look at the usage of AI and cloud, I think it is especially going to accelerate also not just us, but how our clients are going to go on their digital transformation. And I believe this crisis is only going to accelerate that as we go over the next few months."

Arvind Krisna, IBM (2020)

Businesses and organizations with larger, up-to-date resources were able to weather the pandemic, and pivot better than others; one such business was Target (Chopra, 2022). A survey of 22,000 businesses showed an average 29% drop in sales across industries and sizes (with 57% reporting negative impacts due to the pandemic) (Bloom et al., 2021). But that means for over 40% of businesses, the pandemic did not negatively affect profits, whereas some were positively impacted. For most firms, the ability to maintain a presence online or to pivot to offer sales virtually was key to staying open.

These decisions presented differential impacts on businesses, especially small, medium, and single employee businesses. Many small businesses were unable to keep up with the pivot to online delivery of goods and services but were also restricted from physically opening their doors due to the state- and local-level mandates. Government relief programs were introduced to help keep certain businesses afloat, such as funding through the Coronavirus Aid, Relief, and Economic Security (CARES) Act. However, many small and medium businesses were unable to take advantage of this assistance. This is not uncommon during disasters, where many small and medium sized businesses are often more vulnerable (Phillips & Landahl, 2020; Landahl & Neaves 2016; Webb, Tierney, & Dahlhamer, 2000).

The months of March, April, and May in 2020 were when most COVID-19 shutdowns started, as well as social distancing policies.

DOI: 10.1201/9781003319894-5

All states had adopted some form of social distancing measures by March 23 (Adolph et al., 2021). These measures did not begin to relax until May for several states and were more prolonged in many others. Therefore, many of the impacts from them would not have been felt until the second quarter of 2020.

3.1 Technological Impact on Businesses

Prior to the pandemic, many scholars braced for the next evolution in the industrial revolution, known as *Industry 4.0* (Dalenogare et al., 2018; Galanakis et al., 2021; Ghobakhloo, 2020; Lasi et al., 2014). In Industry 4.0, the rapid progression of digital technologies was said to reinvent and reshape the way people work (Ghobakhloo, 2020). Several of the policies, guidelines, and mandates introduced during COVID increased the acceleration of Industry 4.0. Technological innovation during COVID was critical for the continuity of operations in the private sector, especially for small businesses (Abed, 2021). Research and development, supply chain management, and payment systems were all transformed using technology during the pandemic (Almeida et al., 2020). The technologies leveraged include artificial intelligence (AI), big data analytics, blockchain, cloud computing, cyber physical systems (CPS), adaptive manufacturing and the Internet of Things (IoT), mobile devices, and video conferencing software. This was in addition to the plethora of technologies employed in education and healthcare sectors, discussed in Chapters 5 and 7, respectively (Abu Talib et al., 2021; Alabdulaziz, 2021; Alsoufi et al., 2020; Christos Papademetriou et al., 2022; Frank et al., 2021; Fusco et al., 2020; Barman, 2022; Rahman et al., 2022; Shiferaw et al., 2021).

Many research and development labs (from both the private sector and from academia) across all disciplines had to reinvent portions of their experiments and studies during COVID. Whether that was moving to a virtual laboratory environment with collaboration hub tools (e.g., Microsoft Teams), completing studies online with the help of video conferencing tools (e.g., WebEx and Zoom), or installing digital monitoring equipment in physical lab spaces (such as with the use of video cameras or mobile devices) (Kubota, 2021). Qualitative research and non-COVID-related experimental studies were the most challenging, as the virtual space does not easily allow for reading the body language (and other forms of non-verbal communication) of human subject participants. Additionally, non-COVID-related studies did not receive funding for technological-adjustments as COVID-related funding.

Several supply chains had many challenges during the pandemic, including food, manufacturing, and construction. For example, 94% of the Fortune 1000 companies reported issues with their supply chain (Sherman, 2020). Some of the technologies thought to help the supply chain during the pandemic included AI, big data analytics, blockchain, cloud computing, CPS, adaptive manufacturing, and IoT (Acioli et al., 2021; Spieske & Birkel, 2021). The proposed benefits included transparency, competitiveness, and customer satisfaction, among many others (Acioli et al., 2021). In a longitudinal study across industries of supply chain executives, Alicke et al. (2021) found that businesses improved resilience by implementing risk management processes and adopting new practices (Alicke et al., 2021). Success was linked to the adoption of digital technologies, where every industry in their survey invested in advanced analytics. In some instances, remote working contributed to delays in decision-making (Alicke et al. 2021).

There was an increased use of biometric payment systems with facial recognition, fingerprint analysis, or iris identification (Liébana-Cabanillas et al., 2022). Several major credit card companies introduced these security features, widely used during the pandemic (Browne, 2022). Additionally, the use of contactless payments surged (Renu, 2021). This contributed to a rise in e-commerce.

3.1.1 E-Commerce Activities

Online businesses soared during the pandemic; Amazon's profits rose over 220% during COVID (Weise, 2021). In general, e-commerce skyrocketed during the pandemic (Brewster, 2022). However, profits were not evenly distributed among the differing retail trades, even when purchases were made online (Renu, 2021). For example, U.S. retailers saw a significant increase in purchases for building materials and gardening but saw a decline in purchases for clothing and appliances. The impact of COVID on small businesses was devastating;

hundreds of thousands had to shut down (Adam & Alarifi, 2021; Bartik et al., 2020; Segal, 2022).

There were several technological innovations that advanced in the e-commerce space. Several contactless delivery services were introduced, where the customer's goods are ordered and dropped off at selected locations. Contactless payments increased as well. For example, one third-party payment service, PayPal, saw a significant rise in profits amid the pandemic (Hussain, 2021; Renu, 2021). Online entertainment advanced dramatically, as well. Online gaming and digital music concerts offered a safe means of entertainment (Dubois et al., 2022; Renu, 2021).

3.2 Small and Medium Businesses Activities

Small and medium-sized businesses had extraordinary difficulty during the pandemic due to indirect impacts such as a lack of employees, supply chain shortages, and a decline in sales. In general, most studies considered businesses with 20 or more employees as large businesses, while those with four or fewer employees were considered small businesses. For businesses across all sizes, those that were 100% brick and mortar or had face-to-face services, the impact of COVID-19 was more significant than those that could leverage broadband wireless technologies to offer their products through a virtual format (Bloom et al., 2021).

In fact, 43% of small businesses closed – at least temporarily – during the pandemic, putting a strain on finances and local economy (Bartik et al., 2020). One of the most impacted types of businesses was those owned by racial and ethnic minority populations (Baboun, 2020; Bloom et al., 2021; Fairlie, 2020). Minority-owned businesses that remained open experienced a 41% decrease in activity (Fairlie, 2020). This was true even though minority businesses were more likely to add new services to support their employees and community (Dua et al., 2020). Immigrant and women-owned businesses also disproportionally suffered during the pandemic, with a 36% and 25% decrease in activity (Bloom et al., 2021; Fairlie, 2020). These businesses were most likely to have difficulties prior to COVID-19, with limited access to credit and savings (Dua et al., 2020). Hence lending to the Lens of Vulnerability theory mentioned in Chapter 1, where the pre-existing inequities are exacerbated in the wake of a disaster.

The size of the business was not the only factor of concern in determining the impacts of COVID. Nearly every industry group or type was affected during the early months of the pandemic. The agricultural industry had a slight uptick in business owners, while one of the strongest industries – construction – saw a major decline in the first quarter of the pandemic (Fairlie, 2020). Even among essential and non-essential businesses, both saw a decline, though essential businesses had less of a decline (Fairlie, 2020).

The Coronavirus Aid, Relief, and Economic Security (CARES) Act was passed through Congress to help mitigate some of the pressures encountered amid the mandates and restrictions for isolation and social distancing (Katare et al., 2021). For businesses, the primary assistance was through the Paycheck Protection Program (PPP), which could be accessed through the U.S. Small Business Administration (Bartik et al., 2020a, 2020b; Dua et al., 2020; Katare et al., 2021). However, many small businesses did not apply, likely due to the complexity of filling out the forms, bureaucracy, and concerns about eligibility (Bartik et al., 2020a; Dua et al., 2020).

Surviving small businesses were able to change to online sales often used crowdfunding campaigns to secure funds, adjusted how they procured supplies, or increased their social media presence to expand their customer base (Katare et al., 2021). However, there was some indication that not all these adjustments led to a shorter recovery time. In fact, businesses that changed how they procured supplies or served customers experienced a longer recovery time and, in some instances, a loss of income (Katare et al., 2021). Additionally, the use of social media and other online tools to expand the consumer base was correlated with a lower probability of income loss and shortened recovery time (Katare et al., 2021). All of which contributed to more difficulties for smaller businesses, including those who were self-employed.

3.3 Self-Employed Workers

The number of self-employed workers fell by 12%, from 9.3 million workers to 8.2 million workers between February and April 2020

(Kalenkoski, 2020; Kalenkoski & Pablonia, 2020). Most who were self-employed worked from home pre-pandemic and had more flexibility than salary workers (U.S. Bureau of Labor Statistics, 2019).

During the second quarter of 2020, all businesses had difficulties (in terms of profit), none more than businesses with no employees (or those self-employed). The impact on sales during this time period averaged - 40% for those not online and - 30% for online businesses without any employees, mirroring some of the impacts felt by small businesses (Bloom et al., 2021). Travel, art, clothes, and retail industries fared the worst (Bloom et al., 2021).

In a study investigating the initial impact of COVID-19 on employment and hours of unincorporated self-employed workers, Kalenkoski and Pablonia (2020) found differential impacts correlated to gender, marital status, and parental status. Further, the negative impact for April was larger than for March, while there was not much impact from the loosening of restrictions in May. Specifically, marital status and the presence of children were correlated to those who worked, with single people without offspring and married men being able to work longer hours (Kalenkoski & Pablonia, 2020). These results were likely also influenced by school and daycare closures during the pandemic.

There were other impacts for workers due to automation, rapid changes in technology, skill requirements, transitions to low-carbon energy production, and labor (Shutters, 2021). In a comparative study between pre- and post-pandemic predictions on the future of the labor force by 2029, generated through the U.S. Bureau of Labor Statistics, adjustments included an increased demand for skill and knowledge, changes in work shifts, and a reduction in physical labor due to the increased use of technology (Shutters, 2021). Also noted was that changes will be most felt by less educated workers, indicating that there will be a significant decrease in jobs not requiring college-educated workers by 2029. College-educated workers would also shift from non-STEM to STEM-based majors. COVID changed the perception of teleworking, and as such there will be a predicted increased adoption in positions with that flexibility. These predicted changes will likely lead to a reduction of physical job-related injuries, but an increase in illnesses related to sedentary lifestyles.

3.4 Summary

Much more than healthcare, education and work-life were also altered in 2020. The rapid, yet novel, advances in technology allowed e-commerce to thrive while many brick-and-mortar businesses closed. Businesses able to leverage their use of technology to advertise, obtain supplies, and provide services were more likely to recover. Across all industries, larger businesses were more likely to succeed during the pandemic. The strains of social isolation policies especially affected small and medium-sized businesses, predominantly ones that were led by racial and ethnic minorities, women, and immigrants. The preexisting challenges were only exacerbated during the pandemic. Though the use of technology allowed e-commerce to thrive, small and medium-sized businesses across industries did not see the same advances even after incorporating technological adjustments to stay afloat. Furthermore, government interventions such as PPP were largely underutilized by small and medium-sized businesses due to a lack of knowledge about eligibility and the application process.

References

Abed, S. S. (2021). A literature review exploring the role of technology in business survival during the Covid-19 lockdowns. *International Journal of Organizational Analysis, ahead-of-print*(ahead-of-print). https://doi.org/10.1108/IJOA-11-2020-2501

Abu Talib, M., Bettayeb, A. M., & Omer, R. I. (2021). Analytical study on the impact of technology in higher education during the age of COVID-19: Systematic literature review. *Education and Information Technologies, 26*(6), 6719–6746. https://doi.org/10.1007/s10639-021-10507-1

Acioli, C., Scavarda, A., & Reis, A. (2021). Applying industry 4.0 technologies in the COVID–19 sustainable chains. *International Journal of Productivity and Performance Management, 70*(5), 988–1016.

Adam, N. A., & Alarifi, G. (2021). Innovation practices for survival of small and medium enterprises (SMEs) in the COVID-19 times: The role of external support. *Journal of Innovation and Entrepreneurship, 10*(1), 15. https://doi.org/10.1186/s13731-021-00156-6

Adolph, C., Amano, K., Bang-Jensen, B., Fullman, N., & Wilkerson, J. (2021). Pandemic politics: Timing state-level social distancing responses to COVID-19. *Journal of Health Politics, Policy and Law, 46*(2), 211–233. https://doi.org/10.1215/03616878-8802162

Alabdulaziz, M. S. (2021). COVID-19 and the use of digital technology in mathematics education. *Education and Information Technologies, 26*(6), 7609–7633. https://doi.org/10.1007/s10639-021-10602-3

Alicke, K., Barriball, E., & Trautwein, V. (2021, November 23). *How COVID-19 is reshaping supply chains | McKinsey*. Mckinsey and Co. https://www.mckinsey.com/capabilities/operations/our-insights/how-covid-19-is-reshaping-supply-chains

Almeida, F., Santos, J. D., & Monteiro, J. A. (2020). The challenges and opportunities in the digitalization of companies in a post-COVID-19 World. *IEEE Engineering Management Review, 48*(3), 97–103.

Alsoufi, A., Alsuyihili, A., Msherghi, A., Elhadi, A., Atiyah, H., Ashini, A., Ashwieb, A., Ghula, M., Ben Hasan, H., Abudabuos, S., Alameen, H., Abokhdhir, T., Anaiba, M., Nagib, T., Shuwayyah, A., Benothman, R., Arrefae, G., Alkhwayildi, A., Alhadi, A., … Elhadi, M. (2020). Impact of the COVID-19 pandemic on medical education: Medical students' knowledge, attitudes, and practices regarding electronic learning. *PLoS One, 15*(11), e0242905–e0242905. https://doi.org/10.1371/journal.pone.0242905

Baboun, A. (2020, June 22). *The Impact of COVID-19 on minority-owned small businesses in the United States*. Global Resilience Institute. https://globalresilience.northeastern.edu/the-impact-of-covid-19-on-minority-owned-small-businesses-in-the-united-states/

Barman, N. (2022). Digital technology adoption and its impact on the education system during the Covid-19 pandemic. *International Management Review, 18*, 27–92.

Bartik, A., Betrand, M., Cullen, Z. B., Glaeser, E. L., Luca, M., & Stanton, C. T. (2020a). *How are small businesses adjusting to covid-19? Early evidence from a survey [Working Paper]*. National Bureau of Economic Research. https://www.nber.org/system/files/working_papers/w26989/w26989.pdf

Bartik, A. W., Bertrand, M., Cullen, Z., Glaeser, E. L., Luca, M., & Stanton, C. (2020b). The impact of COVID-19 on small business outcomes and expectations. *Proceedings of the National Academy of Sciences, 117*(30), 17656–17666. https://doi.org/10.1073/pnas.2006991117

Bloom, N., Fletcher, R., & Yeh, E. (2021). *Impact of COVID-19 on US Firms [Working paper 28314]*. National Bureau of Economic Research. https://www.nber.org/system/files/working_papers/w28314/w28314.pdf

Brewster, M. (2022, April 27). *E-commerce sales surged during the pandemic*. U.S. Census. https://www.census.gov/library/stories/2022/04/ecommerce-sales-surged-during-pandemic.html

Browne, R. (2022, May 17). *Mastercard launches tech that lets you pay with your face or hand in stores*. CNBC. https://www.cnbc.com/2022/05/17/mastercard-launches-tech-that-lets-you-pay-with-your-face-or-hand.html

Chopra, K. (2022, February 3). What target is doing right in the pandemic era e-commerce race. *Forbes*. https://www.forbes.com/sites/forbestechcouncil/2022/02/03/what-target-is-doing-right-in-the-pandemic-era-e-commerce-race/?sh=5fd83fc13e9e

Dalenogare, L. S., Benitez, G. B., Ayala, N. F., & Frank, A. G. (2018). The expected contribution of industry 4.0 technologies for industrial performance. *International Journal of Production Economics, 204*, 383–394.

Dua, A., Mahajan, D., Millan, I., & Stewart, S. (2020). *COVID-19's effect on minority-owned small businesses | McKinsey.* https://www.mckinsey.com/industries/public-and-social-sector/our-insights/covid-19s-effect-on-minority-owned-small-businesses-in-the-united-states

Dubois, E., Yuan, X., Bennett Gayle, D., Khurana, P., Knight, T., Laforce, S., Turetsky, D., & Wild, D. (2022). Socially vulnerable populations adoption of technology to address lifestyle changes amid COVID-19 in the US. *Data and Information Management, 6*(2), 100001–100001. https://doi.org/10.1016/j.dim.2022.100001

Fairlie, R. (2020). The impact of COVID-19 on small business owners: Evidence from the first three months after widespread social-distancing restrictions. *Journal of Economics & Management Strategy, 29*(4), 727–740. https://doi.org/10.1111/jems.12400

Frank, D.-A., Elbaek, C. T., Borsting, C. K., Mitkidis, P., Otterbring, T., & Borau, S. (2021). Drivers and social implications of artificial intelligence adoption in healthcare during the COVID-19 pandemic. *PLoS One, 16*(11), e0259928–e0259928. https://doi.org/10.1371/journal.pone.0259928

Fusco, A., Dicuonzo, G., Dell'Atti, V., & Tatullo, M. (2020). Blockchain in healthcare: Insights on COVID-19. *International Journal of Environmental Research and Public Health, 17*(19), 1. https://doi.org/10.3390/ijerph17197167

Galanakis, C. M., Rizou, M., Aldawoud, T. M. S., Ucak, I., & Rowan, N. J. (2021). Innovations and technology disruptions in the food sector within the COVID-19 pandemic and post-lockdown era. *Trends in Food Science & Technology, 110*, 193–200. https://doi.org/10.1016/j.tifs.2021.02.002

Ghobakhloo, M. (2020). Industry 4.0, digitization, and opportunities for sustainability. *Journal of Cleaner Production, 252*, 119869. https://doi.org/10.1016/j.jclepro.2019.119869

Hussain, N. (2021, February 3). PayPal profit tops estimates as pandemic drives online spending to record levels. *Reuters.* https://www.reuters.com/article/us-paypal-results-idUSKBN2A332O

Kalenkoski, C., & Pablonia, S. (2020). *Initial Impact of the COVID-19 Pandemic on the Employment and Hours of Self-Employed Coupled and Single Workers by Gender and Parental Status* (No. 48; pp. 741–768). https://www.iza.org/publications/dp/13443/initial-impact-of-the-covid-19-pandemic-on-the-employment-and-hours-of-self-employed-coupled-and-single-workers-by-gender-and-parental-status

Kalenkoski, C. M. (2020). *Differential initial impacts of COVID-19 on the employment and hours of the self-employed* (BLS Working Papers; Working Paper 528). U.S. Department of Labor, U.S. Bureau of Labor Statistics, Office of Productivity and Technology.

Katare, B., Marshall, M. I., & Valdivia, C. B. (2021). Bend or break? Small business survival and strategies during the COVID-19 shock. *International Journal of Disaster Risk Reduction, 61*, 102332. https://doi.org/10.1016/j.ijdrr.2021.102332

Kubota, T. (2021, January 13). Research during the COVID-19 pandemic. *Stanford University News.* https://news.stanford.edu/2021/01/13/research-covid-19-pandemic/

Landahl, M. R., & Neaves, T. T. (2016). Small businesses as a vulnerable population. In *The Future of Disaster Management in the US* (pp. 118–142). Routledge.

Lasi, H., Fettke, P., Kemper, H.-G., Feld, T., & Hoffmann, M. (2014). Industry 4.0. *Business & Information Systems Engineering, 6*(4), 239–242.

Liébana-Cabanillas, F., Muñoz-Leiva, F., Molinillo, S., & Higueras-Castillo, E. (2022). Do biometric payment systems work during the COVID-19 pandemic? Insights from the Spanish users' viewpoint. *Financial Innovation, 8*(1), 22. https://doi.org/10.1186/s40854-021-00328-z

Papademetriou, C., Sofia, A., George, K., & Stylianos, P. (2022). COVID-19 pandemic: The impact of the social media technology on higher education. *Education Sciences, 12*(4), 261. https://doi.org/10.3390/educsci12040261

Phillips, B. D., & Landahl, M. (2020). *Business Continuity Planning: Increasing Workplace Resilience to Disasters.* Butterworth-Heinemann.

Rahman, M. M., Khatun, F., Sami, S. I., & Uzzaman, A. (2022). The evolving roles and impacts of 5G enabled technologies in healthcare: The world epidemic COVID-19 issues. *Array (New York), 14*, 100178–100178. https://doi.org/10.1016/j.array.2022.100178

Renu, N. (2021). Technological advancement in the era of COVID-19. *SAGE Open Medicine, 9*, 20503121211000910. https://doi.org/10.1177/20503121211000912

Segal, E. (2022, January). Covid-related burnout is having a big impact on small business owners: Survey. Forbes. https://www.forbes.com/sites/edwardsegal/2022/01/12/covid-related-burnout-is-having-a-big-impact-on-small-business-owners-survey/

Sherman, E. (2020, February 21). 94% of the fortune 1000 are seeing coronavirus supply chain disruptions. *Fortune.* https://fortune.com/2020/02/21/fortune-1000-coronavirus-china-supply-chain-impact/

Shiferaw, K. B., Mengiste, S. A., Gullslett, M. K., Zeleke, A. A., Tilahun, B., Tebeje, T., Wondimu, R., Desalegn, S., & Mehari, E. A. (2021). Healthcare providers' acceptance of telemedicine and preference of modalities during COVID-19 pandemics in a low-resource setting: An extended UTAUT model. *PLoS One, 16*(4), e0250220–e0250220. https://doi.org/10.1371/journal.pone.0250220

Shutters, S. T. (2021). Modelling long-term COVID-19 impacts on the U.S. workforce of 2029. *PLoS ONE, 16*(12), 1–17. a9h.

Spieske, A., & Birkel, H. (2021). Improving supply chain resilience through industry 4.0: A systematic literature review under the impressions of the COVID-19 pandemic. *Computers & Industrial Engineering, 158*, 107452.

US Bureau of Labor Statistics. (2019). *American Time Use Survey—2021 Results.* https://www.bls.gov/news.release/pdf/atus.pdf

Webb, G. R., Tierney, K. J., & Dahlhamer, J. M. (2000). Businesses and disasters: Empirical patterns and unanswered questions. *Natural Hazards Review, 1*(2), 83–90.

Weise, K. (2021, April 29). Amazon's profit soars 220 percent as pandemic drives shopping online. *The New York Times.* https://www.nytimes.com/2021/04/29/technology/amazons-profits-triple.html

4
EMPLOYMENT DURING COVID-19

"The crisis has uncovered the huge decent work deficits that still prevail in 2020 and shown how vulnerable millions of working people are when a crisis hits."

(Guy Ryder, ILO director general, 2020)

Regardless of the ongoing disaster (or pandemic), for the survivors, daily activities continued. People still had to eat, exercise, and socialize amid the pandemic. What was thought to be a short temporary change in livelihoods turned into nearly two years of social distancing and isolation. Over the longevity of COVID-19, several unique, innovative means to continue daily living outside of work, school, and healthcare were developed. Grocery stores and supermarkets pushed "shop-from-home" options and delivered items to the car. Shopping, in general, moved to curbside delivery of items purchased online. All while, brick-and-mortar facilities remained largely empty.

The pandemic forced employees to work in a completely different environment from what they were used to (Narayanamurthy & Tortorella, 2021). Such policies as social distancing, travel restrictions, wearing masks, and remote work led to behavioral changes in employees – namely the move to a virtual working environment (Gallup, 2020), which in turn affected their emotional, cognitive, and physical well-being (Graves & Karabayeva, 2020). Additionally, the performance of employees was affected while working remotely which led to several concerns, including increased stress, social isolation, burnout, mistrust, and improper infrastructure (Narayanamurthy & Tortorella, 2021; Graves & Karabayeva, 2020). Even building relationships among co-workers and supervisors were negatively impacted by the virtual working environment (Graves & Karabayeva, 2020). In a focus group with a sample of 256 employees (mostly from U.S.

DOI: 10.1201/9781003319894-6

firms), it was reported that 40% of respondents stated that the pandemic would cause fewer cross-functional collaborations, and 36% of the respondents were concerned that remote work might influence the balance of their work and life (Caputo & Hyland, 2020). Williams (2020) noted that the disaster led to an increase in displays of emotions in the workplace, the heightened tensions when people need to struggle with widespread illness, and loss of friends, colleagues, and beloved ones. The pandemic also disrupted household economic stability as millions became unemployed (Lewis and Hsu, 2020; Blustein, Duffy, Ferreira, Cohen-Scali, Cinamon & Allan, 2020). Specifically, work and employment underwent a drastic downturn because of the global pandemic (Matilla-Santander et al., 2021).

Some workers felt working remotely had a positive impact on their employee performance. In one earlier study aptly titled, "Nine Out of Ten (89%) Employees Believe Flexible Working Is Key to Boosting Productivity Levels," found that remote work was more likely to improve the productivity of employees than financial incentives (HSBC, 2017). Furthermore, Stevens (2019) revealed that companies that offer a better work–life balance environment through remote work options can motivate employees and increase worker productivity. This finding was strengthened by Graves and Karabayeva (2020), which reported that remote work increased worker performance, and because of the flexibility it increased the availability of time and access to better talent in the world. And as the pandemic continued on, more and more companies increased their flex options in allowing employees to work from home (at least part-time).

The quick transition to virtual environments during the pandemic tested many of the previous assumptions about job performance, productivity, and profit margins. For some industries, the virtual environments lead to increased profits and better work-life balance for employees. However, amid the pandemic, it became clear that certain segments of employees faced extreme difficulties. For those unable to work remotely, their risk of exposure to the virus was higher than employees who could virtually continue their duties. Disproportionately racial and ethnic minority workers faced unemployment during COVID and in many cases were unable to readily receive uninsurance benefits (Mar et al., 2022). Similarly, these same segments of the population were often employed in jobs, where remote work was not an option, such as essential services (e.g. healthcare, public transportation, custodial, and food service). Similar disparities were found among business owners and self-employed individuals. Fairlie (2020) found that the number of working business owners was reduced by 22% from February to April 2020. Notably, women, minority workers, and workers with precarious employment belong to the group that was most affected globally (Montenovo et al. 2020; Matilla-Santander et al., 2021). As Alon et al. (2020) mentioned, women's employment was focused on service-oriented sectors, the so-called "non-essential" jobs. Furthermore, women, particularly those with young kids, were negatively impacted more than men (Montenovo et al. 2020; Zamarro, Perez-Arce, & Prados, 2020). In addition, African American, immigrant, and female business owners were most influenced by the pandemic because of the shutdown of nonessential activities (Fairlie, 2020), as discussed in Chapter 3. The pandemic classification of workers as essential or non-essential is defined in the next section.

4.1 New Classification of Workers

Amid COVID-19, social distancing guidelines (discussed in Chapter 2) encouraged a classification of businesses and workers. Policies focused on mitigating the spread enacted enforcement of businesses to close if they were deemed non-essential. Businesses determined to be non-essential had to either close temporarily or pivot to a virtual environment for continuity of operations. Digital technologies and digital solutions made it possible for non-essential workers to work in a safe and secure environment.

4.1.1 Essential Workers

Essential workers were individuals who were employed in businesses that were allowed to remain open during the various state- and local-level mandates. Often these businesses and organizations include healthcare employees, grocery store workers, janitorial or custodial staff, public transit workers, among others. Essential workers had an increased opportunity to be exposed to COVID-19 virus. Marginalized groups were overrepresented among essential workers and among non-essential workers furloughed or laid off leading to higher unemployment rates. However, across sectors, various information, and communication technologies (ICT) were introduced to keep essential workers safe.

4.1.1.1 Healthcare

One of the most important segments of essential workers during the pandemic was of those employed in the healthcare industry. As a public health emergency, doctors, nurses, and healthcare providers were critical to managing the threat. Several technologies were adopted by the healthcare industry to minimize exposure to providers and staff. For example, telesurgery and telepharmacy technologies allowed healthcare workers to interact with patients and other providers remotely. Monitoring technologies were introduced, such as digital thermometers and sensors used to identify potentially infected individuals and reduce exposure to healthcare staff. Additionally, artificial intelligence technologies were adopted to maintain health records and serve patients. More information on healthcare technologies is discussed in Chapter 7.

4.1.1.2 Law Enforcement

Law enforcement and related workers, such as firefighters, continued critical in-person tasks during the pandemic. To minimize their exposure, new policies were introduced regarding personal protective measures and interactions with the public. Many of the technologies commonly used prior for law enforcement were hampered during the pandemic. For example, biometrics and surveillance technologies were impaired by many of the public health mitigation measures for COVID. Specifically, the use of masks hindered facial recognition software. The rapid shift in policies and adoption of new technologies, combined with the primary impacts of the pandemic, led to burnout among many law enforcement-related professionals (Clem, 2022; Sener et al. 2021). Clem (2022) examined the impact of burnout (emotional exhaustion, depersonalization, and personal accomplishment) on career commitment to helping professionals (e.g., physicians, law enforcement officers, and clergy) amid the pandemic and found a relationship between burnout and low career commitment.

4.1.1.3 Service Industry

Many aspects of the service industry remained open during the pandemic, namely the food service industry and janitorial services. Technologies were introduced at every stage of the food industry. From food production, slaughterhouses, food processing, and food service (Bhatti et al., 2020; Galanakis et al., 2021; Sharma et al., 2022). Digital tracing tools, data analytics, Internet of Things, robotics, Artificial Intelligence (AI), and e-commerce related apps were used for smart agriculture, supply chain, food security, sustainability, and the safe delivery of services (Galanakis et al., 2021). The tracking of food was accomplished in part by artificial intelligence and the Internet of Things (IoT), as well as blockchain and sensor technology (Sharma et al., 2022). Virtual and augmented reality were employed for remote training of safety measures to reduce the spread of COVID-19 (Galanakis et al., 2021). At the service level, a number of e-commerce apps were used for food delivery and payment, reducing the need for staff (Bhatti et al., 2020).

COVID-19 pandemic-related stressors of being an essential worker influenced not only frontline healthcare workers and first responders, but also low-wage workers, including food and housekeeping/janitorial service workers. Occupational stressors due to COVID-19 experienced by restaurant, food service, and others in low-waged jobs included: (1) fear of being exposed to the virus, (2) working under inadequate safety policies, (3) job insecurity, (4) inconsistent pay and hours, and (5) lack of health benefits or paid time off (Lippert, Furnari, & Kriebel, 2021; Zerden et al. 2022). These contributed to the increased stress and retention of employees (Lippert, Furnari, & Kriebel, 2021; Zerden et al. 2022). In some areas, technologies were used (and developed) specifically for cleaning and reducing the exposure of custodial staff, such as UV radiation, robots, specialized drones to spray disinfectants, and mobile apps to keep track of cleaning duties, among others (Atwell, 2020).

4.1.2 Non-Essential Workers

Non-essential workers were those employed in industries that were forced to physically close, temporarily, or permanently. Among the businesses that temporarily closed, many operated a skeleton crew in their physical locations and virtually provided their services to continue operations. The types of businesses which closed and the length of time they were closed varied by state (and local jurisdiction). However, the workers often considered non-essential included educational staff and faculty, some government employees, and blue-collar workers. Because these businesses closed, those unable to afford to maintain all staff decided to furlough or lay off some employees. This led to a significant spike in unemployment across the U.S. Information about the impacts on businesses were discussed in Chapter 3.

4.1.2.1 Education

During the pandemic, teachers, schools, and districts needed to transform their curriculum and pedagogy from face-to-face to virtual, then to hybrid, and finally face-to-face again. The technologies leveraged included broadband wireless technologies, such as video conferencing, learning management systems, and discipline-specific software. The adoption of these technologies contributed to some of the challenges. For example, some teachers struggled to adopt new teaching approaches (Honigsfeld & Nordmeyer, 2020) or adopt new technology platforms (Wiggins, 2020), which contributed to higher levels of stress (Pressley, 2021). Also, the willingness to adopt new digital teaching platforms may have adversely affected evaluations. In a study with 361 participants to explore how the new teaching approaches and requirements had influenced teachers' self-efficacy (e.g., instructional and engagement efficacy), results indicated that teachers who were teaching virtually had the lowest efficacy scores in comparison to teachers in a hybrid or in-person modalities (Pressley, & Ha, 2021). While teachers faced many concerns with temporary remote teaching, students and parents were also affected as discussed in Chapter 5.

4.1.2.2 Service Industry

The service industry was unique in that some businesses fell into essential status while others were deemed non-essential. For example, the sudden lock down due to the outbreak of COVID-19 and the digital work connectivity caused challenges in the hospitality industry (Hunt, 2020; Hao et al., 2020; Ren & Chadee, 2019), including self-control depletion, and disengagement from work (Chadee, Ren, & Tang, 2021). Women and younger hospitality employees may have had disproportionate impacts (Chen 2021). As mentioned by Chadee, Ren, and Tang (2021), although many hospitality units were closed during the pandemic, employers and back-office employees continued to work remotely to keep the business running. The outcome was the creation of a new normal for employees in hospitality and service industries to use telework technologies, other technologies introduced were previously mentioned under the essential worker section of this chapter.

4.1.2.3 Unemployment

As non-essential businesses closed their physical locations, they reduced staff. Previously working in precarious and non-unionized jobs, during the pandemic many of these employees were laid off. According to Matilla-Santander et al. (2021), those employed in precarious jobs often found themselves in situations where they worked under threat of exposure due to insufficient social and health protections and did not qualify for government assistance. To some extent, precarious employment was an important social determinant of health that disproportionately impacted marginalized populations and contributed to adverse health outcomes. Precarious employment issues are likely to cause substance use disorders, and mental health issues including suicidal tendencies (Matilla-Santander et al., 2021).

However, in some businesses, the adoption of technology contributed to forced layoffs and furloughs, as robots, automation, and mobile technology with assistance from AI were introduced (Parvez et al., 2022). The unemployment situation was thought to be exacerbated due to the growth of digitalization (International Labor Organization, 2020). The total impact of technology on unemployment has yet to be fully explored. Some argued that increased use of ICT for business continuity reduced layoffs during the pandemic (Pierri & Timmer, 2020).

In any case, the combination of precarious employment and increased use of digital technologies led to massive unemployment. During the second quarter of 2020, at the height of the pandemic and subsequent social distancing policies in the U.S., the unemployment rate was as high as 13% (Smith et al. 2021). The unemployment rate was higher for some demographics, such as Hispanic/Latino, African American, Asian and women workers, at 17%, 16.3%, 14.4%, and 14.1% respectively (Smith et al., 2021; Karpman, Gonzalez, & Kenney, 2020). Hispanics with non-citizen family members also reported increased unemployment or reduced work hours (Gonzalez et al., 2020). Some provided pre-warning of the vulnerability of young people in the workforce before and during the pandemic (International Labor Organization, 2020; Blustein et al. 2020).

4.1.2.4 Working from Home

The pandemic caused many to lose jobs, but it offered opportunities for workers to work from home, which to a large extent dampened the economic crisis (Barrero, Bloom, & Davis, 2020; Bick, Blandin, & Mertens 2020; Kalenkoski, & Pabilonia, 2020b), and "become the magic bullet for enabling large segments of society to function" (Rivera, 2020). As mentioned by Wright, Riemann, and Fisher (2022), many people experienced some degree of work-life imbalance during the COVID-19 restrictions in the U.S. (from March to June 2020) because they had to spend more time at home to earn a living (Viner et al., 2020). Researchers reported that new communication technologies may have improved work-life balance for some people, especially when they realized that these technologies would give them increased flexibility (Brough et al., 2020). However, some technologies used for telework employees were able to monitor productivity and surveillance (Newlands et al., 2020; Vitak & Zimmer, 2021).

However, as Kossek and Ozeki (1998) mentioned, when work obligations interfere with family responsibilities or family responsibilities interfere with work obligations, work-life imbalance occurred. Work-life imbalance (and use of technology for work) may lead to increased stress and burnout, higher absenteeism, substance abuse disorders, worker turnover intentions, physical health issues, and job dissatisfaction (Martins et al., 2002; Lee & Sirgy, 2019). Mentioned in Chapter 3, the woman burdened with working from home and being primary home care providers for young children, the stress was unbearable (Census Bureau, 2020). In a study investigating how COVID-19 influenced parents' labor supply, Heggeness (2020) found that working mothers in states where stay-at-home orders and school closures were executed early were 68.8% more likely to take leave from their jobs than those in states where closures were operated later. For those mothers who chose to continue working, they worked more hours than comparable fathers (Heggeness, 2020). These results indicate that women were vulnerable to disasters in terms of career growth. This contributed to a mass exodus of women in the labor market globally (Bateman & Ross, 2020; Gonzales, 2022).

4.2 Summary

This chapter discusses the adoption of technology by and for workers during the pandemic, both essential and non-essential workers in the U.S. Several technological innovations were leveraged across industry including, monitoring technology, sensors, digital thermometers, artificial intelligence, surveillance technologies, biometrics, digital tracing, Internet of Things, e-commerce apps, data analytics, blockchain technology, video conferencing, learning management systems, computers, and mobile devices. The inequity issues were worsened among the vulnerable groups because of the disparities caused by the pandemic. Racial and ethnic minorities and women were overrepresented in essential jobs, increasing their exposure. Simultaneously, racial and ethnic minorities and women were unemployed at high rates, in non-essential jobs. In non-essential jobs, precarious work environments and the increase of digitization may have contributed to the higher unemployment rates globally. This calls for policymakers and administrative staff to understand the needs of the said populations in the future to create policies and guidelines that consider the various needs.

References

Alon, T. M., Doepke, M., Olmstead-Rumsey, J., & Tertilt, M. (2020). The Impact of COVID-19 on Gender Equality. NBER Working Paper No. 26947.

Atwell, C. (2020). Top 6 cleaning technologies during COVID-19. *EETimes.* https://www.eetimes.com/top-6-new-cleaning-technologies-implemented-during-the-pandemic/

Barrero, J. M., Bloom, N., & Davis, S. J. (2020). COVID-19 is also a reallocation shock. *Brookings Papers on Economic Activity.*

Bick, A., Blandin, A., & Mertens, K. (2020). Work from Home after the COVID-19 Outbreak. Federal Reserve Bank of Dallas Research Department Working Papers. https://doi.org10.24149/wp2017

Blustein, D. L., Duffy, R., Ferreira, J. A., Cohen-Scali, V., Cinamon, R. G., & Allan, B. A. (2020). Unemployment in the time of COVID-19: A research agenda. *Journal of Vocational Behavior, 119*, 1034.

Brough, P., Timms, C., Chan, X. W., Hawkes, A., & Rasmussen, L. (2020). Work–life balance: Definitions, causes, and consequences. In T. Theorell (Ed.), *Handbook of socioeconomic determinants of occupational health: From macro-level to micro-level evidence* (pp. 473–487). Springer.

Caputo, A., & Hyland, P. (2020). Employee concerns about COVID-19. https://www.mmc.com/insights/publications/2020/march/employee-concerns-about-covid-19.html. Accessed on July 1, 2020.

Census Bureau, U. S. (2020). *Working Moms Bear Brunt of Home Schooling While Working During COVID-19*. https://www.census.gov/library/stories/2020/08/parents-juggle-work-and-child-care-during-pandemic.html

Chadee, D., Ren, S., & Tang, G. (2021). Is digital technology the magic bullet for performing work at home? Lessons learned for post COVID-19 recovery in hospitality management. *International Journal of Hospitality Management, 92*, 102718.

Chen, M. H. (2021). Well-being and career change intention: COVID-19's impact on unemployed and furloughed hospitality workers. *International Journal of Contemporary Hospitality Management, 33*(8), 2500–2520.

Clem, C. L. (2022). The Impact of Burnout on Career Commitment Among Physicians, Clergy, and Law Enforcement During the COVID-19 Pandemic: A Quantitative Study.

Fairlie, R. W. (2020). The Impact of COVID-19 on Small Business Owners: Evidence of Early-Stage Losses from the April 2020 Current Population Survey. IZA Discussion Paper No. 13311.

Families First Coronavirus Response Act. (2020). Families first coronavirus response act: Employee paid leave rights. US Department of Labor. https://www.dol.gov/agencies/whd/pandemic/ffcra-employee-paid-leave. Accessed on May 18, 2020.

Gallup. (2020, April 7). How leaders are responding to COVID-19 workplace disruption. https://www.gallup.com/workplace/307622/leaders-responding-co vid-workplace-disruption.aspx. Accessed on July 1, 2020.

Gonzalez, D., Karpman, M., Kenney, G. M., & Zuckerman, S. (2020). *Hispanic adults in families with noncitizens disproportionately feel the economic fallout from COVID-19*. Urban Institute.

Graves, L., & Karabayeva, A. (2020). Managing virtual workers-strategies for success. *IEEE Engineering Management Review, 48*(2), 166–172.

Hao, F., Xiao, Q., & Chon, K. (2020). COVID-19 and China's hotel industry: Impacts, a disaster management framework, and post-pandemic agenda. *International Journal of Hospitality Management, 90*, 102636.

Heggeness, M. L. (2020). Why is Mommy so stressed? Estimating the immediate impact of the covid-19 shock on parental attachment to the labor market and the double bind of mothers. Opportunity and Inclusive Growth Institute, Federal Reserve Bank of Minnesota, Institute Working Paper, (33).

Honigsfeld, A., & Nordmeyer, J. (2020). Teacher collaboration during a global pandemic *Educational Leadership* [Special report]. http://www.ascd.org/publications/educational-leadership/summer20/vol77/num10/Teacher-Collaboration-During-a-Global-Pandemic.aspx, 77, 47, 50.

HSBC. (2017). Nine out of ten (89%) employees believe flexible working is key to boosting productivity levels. https://www.google.co.uk/url?sa=t&rct=j&q=&esrc=s&source=web&cd=2&ved=2ahUKEwiDlPj01rDpAhXDURUIHY0_BsUQFjABegQIChAE&url=https%3A%2F%2Fwww.about.hsbc.co.uk%2F-%2Fmedia%2Fuk%2Fen%2Fnews-

and-media%2Fcmb%2F171108-flexible-working.pdf&usg=AOvVaw
35r5jxp67zZU1_oBQUo4B0. Accessed July 1, 2020.
Hunt, R. (2020). Marriott CEO: Coronavirus is hurting the hotel chain worse
than 9/11 or World War II. https://www.nasdaq.com/articles/marriott-
ceo%3A-coronavirus-is-hurting-the-hotel-chain-worse-than-9-11-or-
world-war-ii-2020. Accessed on March 25, 2020.
International Labor Organization.(2020). *Policy brief: The world of work and
COVID-19.* United Nations.
Kalenkoski, C. M., & Pabilonia, S. W. (2020b). Initial impact of the COVID-19
pandemic on the employment and hours of self-employed coupled and
single workers by gender and parental status.
Karpman, M., Gonzalez, D., & Kenney, G. M. (2020). *Parents are struggling to
provide for their families during the pandemic.* Urban Institute.
Kossek, E., & Ozeki, C. (1998). Work–family conflict, policies, and the job–
life satisfaction relationship: A review and directions for organizational
behavior–human resources research. *Journal of Applied Psychology, 83*(2), 139.
Lee, D. J., & Sirgy, M. J. (2019). Work-life balance in the digital workplace: The
impact of schedule flexibility and telecommuting on work-life balance and
overall life satisfaction. In M. Coetzee (Ed.), *Thriving in digital workspaces*
(pp. 355–384). Springer.
Lewis, B., & T. Hsu (2020). The collateral damage of the coronavirus.
https://www.nytimes.com/2020/05/09/business/economy/coronavirus-
unemployment.html. Accessed on May 10, 2020.
Lippert, J. F., Furnari, M. B., & Kriebel, C. W. (2021). The impact of the Covid-19
pandemic on occupational stress in restaurant work: A qualitative study.
International Journal of Environmental Research and Public Health, 18(19), 10378.
Martins, L. L., Eddleston, K. A., & Veiga, J. F. (2002). Moderators of the relationship between work-family conflict and career satisfaction. *Academy
of Management Journal, 45*(2), 399–409. https://doi.org/libproxy.albany.
edu/10.5465/3069354
Matilla-Santander, N., Ahonen, E., Albin, M., Baron, S., Bolíbar, M., Bosmans,
K., ... & All Members of the PWR Study Consortium. (2021). COVID-19
and precarious employment: consequences of the evolving crisis. *Interna-
tional Journal of Health Services, 51*(2), 226–228.
Montenovo, L., Jiang, X., Rojoas, F. L., Schmutte, I. M., Simon, K. I., Weinberg,
B. A., & Wing, C. (2020). Determinants of Disparities in COVID-19 Job
Losses. NBER Working Paper No. 21732.
Narayanamurthy, G., & Tortorella, G. (2021). Impact of COVID-19 outbreak
on employee performance–moderating role of industry 4.0 base technolo-
gies. *International Journal of Production Economics, 234*, 108075.
Newlands, G., Lutz, C., Tamò-Larrieux, A., Villaronga, E. F., Harasgama,
R., & Scheitlin, G. (2020). Innovation under pressure: Implications
for data privacy during the Covid-19 pandemic. *Big Data & Society, 7*(2),
2053951720976680. https://doi.org/10.1177/2053951720976680
Pressley, T. (2021). Factors contributing to teacher burnout during COVID-19.
Educational Researcher, 50(5), 325–327. https://doi.org/10.3102/00131
89X211004138

Pressley, T., & Ha, C. (2021). Teaching during a pandemic: United States teachers' self-efficacy during COVID-19. *Teaching and Teacher Education*, *106*, 103465.

Ren, S., & Chadee, D., 2019. Influence of guanxi on hospitality career performance in China: Is more necessarily better? *International Journal of Hospitality Management*. https://doi.org/10.1016/j.ijhm.2019.102420 in press.

Rivera, M. A. (2020). Hitting the reset button for hospitality research in times of crisis: Covid19 and beyond. *International Journal of Hospitality Management*, *87*. https://doi.org/10.1016/j.ijhm.2020.102528

Sener, H., Arikan, I., Gündüz, N., & Gülekci, Y. (2021). Detecting the relationship between the stress levels and perceived burnout in law-enforcement officers during the COVID-19 outbreak: A cross-sectional study. *Social Work in Public Health*, *36*(4), 486–495.

Smith, S., Edwards, R., & Duong, H., (2021). *Unemployment rises in 2020, as the country battles the COVID-19 pandemic*. US Bureau of Labor Statistics: Monthly Labor Review. https://www.bls.gov/opub/mlr/2021/article/unemployment-rises-in-2020-as-the-country-battles-the-covid-19-pandemic.htm. Accessed on October 30, 2022.

Stevens, P., 2019. The 2019 flexible working survey. Wildgoose. https://wearewildgoose.com/uk/news/flexible-working-survey-insights/. Accessed on July 1, 2020.

Viner, R. M., Russell, S., Croker, H., Packer, J., Ward, J., Stansfield, C., Mytton, O., Bonell, C., & Booy, R. (2020). School closure and management practices during coronavirus outbreaks including COVID-19: A rapid systematic review. *The Lancet Child & Adolescent Health*, *4*(5). 397–404.

Vitak, J., & Zimmer, M. (2021). Workers' attitudes toward Increased Surveillance during and after the Covid-19 Pandemic. *Items: Insights from the Social Sciences*.

Wiggins, A. (2020). A brave new world: A teacher's take on surviving distance learning

Williams, M. (2020, May 19). Coronavirus class divide – the jobs most at risk of contracting and dying from COVID-19. *The Conversation*. https://theconversation.com/coronavirus-class-divide-the-jobs-most-at-risk-of-contracting-and-dying-from-covid-19-138857. Accessed on May, 20 2020.

Wright, K. B., Riemann, W., & Fisher, C. L. (2022). Work–life-imbalance during the COVID-19 pandemic: exploring social support and health outcomes in the United States. *Journal of Applied Communication Research*, *50*(1), 54–69.

Zamarro, G. F., Perez-Arce, F., & Prados, M. J. (2020). Gender Differences in the Impact of COVID-19." Working Paper. https://tinyurl.com/CESRGenderDiffs

Zerden, L. D. S., Richman, E. L., Lombardi, B., & Forte, A. B. (2022). Frontline, essential, and invisible: The needs of low-wage workers in hospital settings during COVID-19. *Workplace Health & Safety*, *70*(11), 509–514. https://doi.org/10.1177/21650799221108490

5
EDUCATION DURING COVID-19

"The convenience of being able to wake up and log into class was one of the most surprising things about virtual learning. It allowed me to expand the number of activities... But this also meant I would be online for 12 hours a day. That was really difficult for me."

(Denis Alvarez, College student (Richards et al., 2021))

The pandemic significantly altered how we learned in the U.S., from K-12 to postsecondary education. The guidance to stay home to reduce the spread of the virus also meant that our schools and institutes of higher education (IHEs) closed their physical doors. Instead, most adjusted to temporary remote education, typically with the assistance of computers, the internet, video conferencing tools, and online learning management systems. Globally, more than 90% of the students enrolled were subjected to school closures (Jalongo, 2021). This chapter briefly outlines the government guidance provided to public education systems (K-12 and IHEs), the variation in impacts for different populations, and the impact of changes to education during COVID-19.

The shift to online instruction contributed to increased marginalization, pressure on families, stress for teachers, interruption of learning, and the reevaluation of the digital divide and literacy, as well as innovative technological solutions to learning while socially distant (Jalongo, 2021). For millions of children, young adults, and individuals pursuing higher education, schools and libraries were the primary means of connecting to the internet. However, as schools closed and moved to remote education, these students had to remain at home to complete their homework, participate in class discussions, and adapt to the online testing environment. This shift also set the bar for technological

DOI: 10.1201/9781003319894-7

innovations in how education was taught, and learning was facilitated. Many had to adapt to changes, and institutions quickly valued the importance of investing in quality systems and software to guarantee continuity of operations awareness (Panja & Choudhury, 2022).

5.1 Educational Guidance

The guidance to reduce the marginalization of students and teachers, and how to best offer support from the educational entities, was not always clear. At the federal level, there were snippets of information provided through the US Department of Education (Dept of Ed) and the Centers for Disease Control and Prevention (CDC), while much of the guidance was again pushed through state-level entities. Most of the state-level guidance recommended learning support during school closures, with variations on how to provide such support. Though, many students relied on schools to provide much more than just an education, therefore guidance encouraged schools to plan to provide support for other needs, such as food, mental health, and other social services (Reich et al., 2020). The guidance also mentioned considerations for vulnerable populations, such as students with disabilities and students for whom English is a second language. However, these considerations were not standardized across states and, in some cases, not specific within the state. For example, while nearly every state included considerations for people with disabilities, only some had plans regarding language development and regarding students for whom English was a second language.

At the K-12 level, all 50 states provided a waiver to bypass state assessments. Similarly, many IHEs waived standardized testing requirements for undergraduate and graduate programs, with variations occurring per institution and even per program. Most IHEs offered temporary remote online instructions. Again, some universities and colleges were aware of the other needs of students, such as housing, technology, food, and health services (including mental), and therefore incorporated plans to loan technology, facilitate quarantine housing, continue food pantries, etc. However, such considerations varied across institutions. This was an important consideration for IHEs as many college students faced homelessness and food inequities (Broton, 2020; Hallett & Freas, 2018; Haskett et al., 2020; Winkle-Wagner, 2009).

The lack of preparedness and proper guidance for such a prolonged disaster situation forced many permanent school closures, mergers, and reorganizations. The protracted length of the pandemic also caused many schools and governments to rush to return to normalcy as quickly as possible. However, the return to in-person (and hybrid) instruction was correlated with an increase in cases and deaths and was more significant in counties without mask mandates (Chernozhukov et al., 2021). After a year of remote instruction, most IHEs returned, at least in part, to in-person classes. Once reopened, many had guidance around masks, testing, and on isolation, once vaccines became available, universities and colleges implemented policies for that as well (Mossa-Basha et al., 2020).

5.2 Digital Divide in Education

The digital divide, as defined in Chapter 1, focused on the gap between those with access to broadband wireless technologies and those without, leaving many segments of the population disadvantaged (Cullen, 2001; van Dijk, 2006). However, it is also about equitable access to these technologies (Gorski, 2005). In the educational context, this gap has been seen in primary, secondary, and postsecondary education (Buzzetto-Hollywood, 2021). Inaccessible technology had broader implications regarding equitable access to education and the ability to gain knowledge. Some students did not have access to technologies (Simmons, 2020). These inequities impacted the most marginalized, such as those experiencing homelessness and low-income populations, among others. Prior to the pandemic, K-12 school systems increasingly used broadband wireless technologies for instruction and to reach parents. Similarly, universities and other IHEs had expanded their use of technology, offering coursework fully online. However, at the time of the pandemic, most instruction at all levels of education was still offered in face-to-face formats. Even at most universities that offered some coursework or entire degree programs online, most of the majors' curricula were offered in person. While inequities due to the digital divide were acknowledged pre-pandemic, the impacts were more pronounced during the pandemic because of the near ubiquitous use of broadband wireless-based devices and systems for education.

5.3 Educational Impacts During COVID-19

The shift to online education and remote learning with little standardization led to a variety of impacts on students, parents, and teachers – at all levels of education. Even the impact of the pandemic on childcare was significant, with many closings due to parents working from home.

Bansak and Starr (2021) carried out a study to assess the sudden shift to distance learning using data from US Census Bureau's Household Pulse Survey. They found that parents and children consumed significantly more time in learning activities when their schools offered multiple educational support. As shown in Figure 5.1, the shift to remote learning likely varied across states, where the range of households reporting was from 47% to 86%. Teacher contact was less than 55% for many households with some northeastern and western states showing a higher percentage. Problems with the devices or accessibility to the internet were as high as 31% in some states, based on household reporting, in which Louisiana and Mississippi households experienced the brunt of the impacts. Finally, Figure 5.1 also shows the percentage of households reporting an increased burden on parents to assist in the teaching activities with their students, with as many as 83% of households reporting this in some states.

Therefore, this section discusses the use of technology for education, learning, and childcare below. The topical areas are further segmented based on the age-related institutional structures in the U.S.: (1) Childcare (generally for children three and under); (2) Pre-K to 12th grade (in general for children between 3 and 18), and (3) IHEs (for those interested in postsecondary education often 18 and older).

5.3.1 Childcare

Home-based childcare centers saw a boom sparking innovative technological solutions to help connect potential clients to providers (Luscombe, 2020). Parents felt the impact of having children being educated at home. Everything from software for learning, social connection, and exercise were readily shared with parents struggling to juggle childcare and work from home (McQuate, 2020). This proved to be a burden for many parents. Approximately 20% of parents

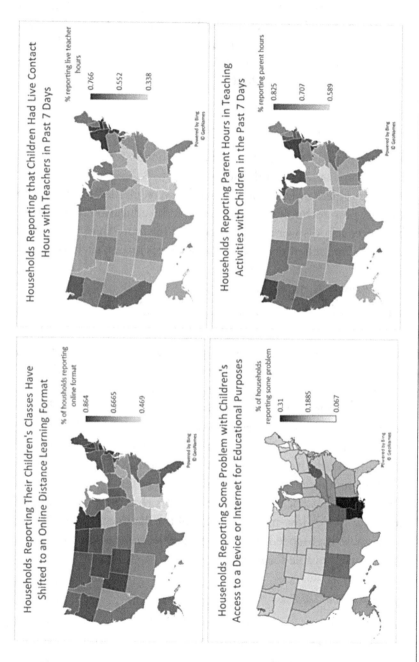

Figure 5.1 Geographic variation related to shocks in education. (Source: Bansak & Starr, 2021.)

stopped working due to childcare issues, though a majority of the burden fell on working mothers (Bureau, 2020) and contributed to a significant decline in women in the labor force (Bateman & Ross, 2020; Fry, 2022; Gonzales, 2022). The brunt of the responsibility fell on parents, greatest for those with pre-K, elementary, or students with disabilities (Slavin & Storey, 2020).

5.3.2 Pre-K to 12th Grade

The pivot to remote online instruction, even though temporary, caused anxiety for some students and teachers (Gupta & Jawanda, 2020, p2). Students struggled to learn, and teachers were challenged with the adoption of new technologies and systems for educational activities. Furthermore, schools were often important for more than just course instruction, some relied on schools for other resources, such as food.

5.3.2.1 Impacts on Learning

Secondary impacts from the use of technology for education included "increased health issues from being inside, social isolation, addiction to internet/social media, increased risk of child exploitation, increased risk due to intersectionality[1] (such as children with disabilities)" (Gupta & Jawanda, 2020). Many of the barriers explored internationally were related to the inaccessibility of broadband wireless or devices to pursue remote education, which was connected to family income (Abu Talib et al., 2021; Alsoufi et al., 2020). There is evidence that this inaccessibility was also related to family income domestically. Implementation of remote education was better in areas with high-SES school districts, and worse in areas that cater to racial and ethnic minorities or low-income households (Slavin & Storey, 2020). Without stable high-speed internet service, learning remotely would have been unachievable for many.

5.3.2.2 Impacts on Teachers

The impact on teachers was unprecedented. The forced pedagogical innovation provided more flexibility (Abu Talib et al., 2021; Mustapha et al., 2021). Early education teachers, despite any barriers, successfully adapted to remote online instruction of children 2 to 5 years old

(McKenna et al., 2021). However, the transition to temporary remote learning caused significant stress, additional workload, and low morale for teachers and academic staff, forced to shift so rapidly (Abu Talib et al., 2021; Alsoufi et al., 2020; Hall-Mills et al., 2022). And some teachers struggled to provide online instruction (Slavin & Storey, 2020). A few of the challenges noted were issues engaging students, meeting with parents, a few guidelines, and various levels of internet and computer access for students (Francom et al., 2021). Several studies presented options on how to improve teacher preparedness for future incidents. The options included clear plans and communication for emergencies and incorporating online components and training within current face-to-face classes and professional development for online learning, technology access, and technology training for both teachers and students (An et al., 2021; Francom et al., 2021). When teachers were unable to effectively use devices and software for remote instruction, they were unable to provide the most robust and appropriately rigorous curricula. This impacted student learning and knowledge.

5.3.2.3 Access to Other Resources

Some students were disadvantaged beyond their technological access. For example, students experiencing homelessness may have had additional needs, such as food, healthcare, and social support previously obtained at school (Slavin & Storey, 2020). As mentioned earlier, considerations for these types of accommodations were not universal across all school districts. Schools offering devices noticed there was a potential for a lack of access to broadband wireless technologies to fully utilize internet-based software (Slavin & Storey, 2020).

5.3.3 Colleges and Universities

5.3.3.1 Students

There were varying impacts among college students. Some students excelled, such as those eager to proceed at their own pace. Similarly, those with discomfort or anxiety with face-to-face communication could thrive with the variety of discussion opportunities online, and students were exposed to modern technologies (Abu Talib et al., 2021). However, some students were disadvantaged in terms of having equal access to education due to their household access to Wi-Fi, finding a quiet space in the home, or their digital literacy. Student participation, engagement, and motivation suffered due to fatigue, stress, boredom, and isolation (Abu Talib et al., 2021). Additionally, the direct impacts of the pandemic weighed on the hearts and minds of adult students at IHES, disproportionately on marginalized students. A study of over 2,500 college students reported that higher stress and mental health risks were found among women, non-Hispanic Asian, in fair/poor health, of below-average relative family income, or who knew someone infected with COVID-19 (Browning et al., 2021).

5.3.3.2 Professors

Professors were also similarly stressed by the direct impacts and the rapid shift to online education (Abu Talib et al., 2021; Crawford & Simon, 2021). Digital literacy also varied among professors, causing additional struggles with instruction. Building necessary relationships between professors and students, or among students was difficult in the online format. This had an impact on student engagement and participation (Abu Talib et al., 2021). However, remote learning offered convenience and flexibility, not often possible before. The push online forced change and innovation, exposed problems, reduced costs, and created exposure to technology among underserved populations (Abu Talib et al., 2021).

5.3.3.3 Access to Resources

IHEs often offered more than just education. In the same way K-12 students relied on school for other resources such as hot meals and access to Wi-Fi. College students mostly lived, ate, socialized, and used the libraries on campus (Altman, 2022), and often found themselves reliant on IHEs for more than just education. The rapid pivot to temporary remote instruction was devastating to college students, not just for their educational needs but for their living arrangements, as well. As colleges and universities changed to remote instruction, they simultaneously closed physical infrastructure on campuses, including dormitories, dining halls, student centers, and some libraries. Though some campuses used this time as an opportunity to test new innovations related to technology, such as robots used for food delivery at George Mason University (Black, 2020; Williams, 2020).

Despite the potential for new innovated methods of offering extended resources, there is evidence that the changes during the pandemic contributed to their overall mental health (Browning et al., 2021; Lederer et al., 2021; Son et al., 2020; Wang et al., 2020). With the increased housing and food insecurity among the collegiate populations, quick shifts during the pandemic left many students facing homelessness (Lederer et al., 2021). Access to technology may have been a priority, but no bigger priority than trying to determine where and in which quiet space some students might have to use said technology. Again, these issues challenged racial and ethnic minority students more than others (Lederer et al., 2021).

5.4 Challenges across Academic Levels

5.4.1 Technology-Associated Systemic Inequities

The use of technologies not universally accessible further complicated matters for many students at all academic levels. For example, students with disabilities felt further marginalized, with reported issues and discomfort with the technology required for remote learning (Schafer et al., 2021). Students and families for low-income households were challenged with having proper access to broadband wireless, which often carries an increased cost, where poor internet bandwidth and other technical difficulties caused problems with the flow of communication for online courses (Abu Talib et al., 2021). In some ways, there were technology-associated systemic inequities, often seen associated with marginalized communities, following preexisting challenges with the digital divide and equity (Moldavan et al., 2022).

5.4.2 Digital and Technical Literacy

Furthermore, digital and technical literacy varied from person to person among students, parents, and administrative staff (Abu Talib et al., 2021). This impacted the success of the courses and of those learning. An unspoken assumption built into the shift to temporary remote instruction was that most people were technically savvy enough to make the quick change or that they could get the necessary assistance from someone in their quarantine pod (or household). Many who lacked digital literacy were left without assistance at home, and there were few thoughtful technological training opportunities offered through their schools, remotely.

5.4.3 Course Type

The move to online learning was also not universally rigorous or robust for all types of courses. Some coursework was not easily instructed through online remote instruction, because the technology was not adequate (Abu Talib et al., 2021). Students and faculty from STEM-related fields had problems using the online systems, such as the medical field (Abu Talib et al., 2021; Mustapha et al., 2021). Within fields that were heavy on mathematics, some studies show that the pivot to online instruction increased anxiety and mental health concerns for students (Lanius et al., 2022). Other curricula were challenged as well. Physical education teachers found frustration with the move to remote education and the marginalization of the subject matter by administrators (J. Johnson et al., 2021). Similarly, this challenged many directors for band class and other music-based instruction (Hash, 2021). Although evidence from a study in China indicated that many students and teachers were comfortable with chemistry taught through online instruction with virtual experiments, given use of the proper software (Huang, 2020).

5.5 Summary

The response to the pandemic significantly impacted education and learning for students of all age groups. For students under 18, the change also affected their parents and general household. Childcare was a concern for parents who were working from home, with most of the burden on working mothers, who in turn dropped from the workforce at an alarming rate. From elementary school to postsecondary education, the reliance on technology had unintended consequences including increased mental health issues and social isolation. The stressors were faced by students, parents, and teachers. Furthermore, in most instances, the reliance on technology was solely focused on replacing in-person instruction, with less attention paid to the other resources needed by students often found at school, such as food, housing, and socialization. Again, the stressors were most often felt by traditionally marginalized groups, including women, racial/ethnic minorities, students with disabilities, and low-income populations.

Note

1 A term coined by Kimberlé Crenshaw to address the multiple identities (social forces) which impact power and access, often where disadvantages are legitimized. (Crenshaw 2017).

References

Abu Talib, M., Bettayeb, A. M., & Omer, R. I. (2021). Analytical study on the impact of technology in higher education during the age of COVID-19: Systematic literature review. *Education and Information Technologies, 26*(6), 6719–6746. https://doi.org/10.1007/s10639-021-10507-1

Alsoufi, A., Alsuyihili, A., Msherghi, A., Elhadi, A., Atiyah, H., Ashini, A., Ashwieb, A., Ghula, M., Ben Hasan, H., Abudabuos, S., Alameen, H., Abokhdhir, T., Anaiba, M., Nagib, T., Shuwayyah, A., Benothman, R., Arrefae, G., Alkhwayildi, A., Alhadi, A., … Elhadi, M. (2020). Impact of the COVID-19 pandemic on medical education: Medical students' knowledge, attitudes, and practices regarding electronic learning. *PLoS One, 15*(11), e0242905. https://doi.org/10.1371/journal.pone.0242905

Altman, A. (2022). Library technology and its perceptions at small institutions of higher education: The COVID-19 factor. *Journal of Library Administration, 62*(1), 67–84. a9h.

An, Y., Kaplan-Rakowski, R., Yang, J., Conan, J., Kinard, W., & Daughrity, L. (2021). Examining K-12 teachers' feelings, experiences, and perspectives regarding online teaching during the early stage of the COVID-19 pandemic. *Educational Technology Research & Development, 69*(5), 2589–2613. a9h.

Bansak, C., & Starr, M. (2021). Covid-19 shocks to education supply: How 200,000 U.S. households dealt with the sudden shift to distance learning. *Review of Economics of the Household, 19*(1), 63–90. https://doi.org/10.1007/s11150-020-09540-9

Bateman, N., & Ross, M. (2020). *Why has COVID-19 been especially harmful for working women?* Brookings. https://www.brookings.edu/essay/why-has-covid-19-been-especially-harmful-for-working-women/

Black, J. (2020, July 13). With robot deliveries and outdoor tents, campus dining will be very different. *The New York Times.* https://www.nytimes.com/2020/07/13/dining/college-food-coronavirus.html

Broton, K. M. (2020). A review of estimates of housing insecurity and homelessness among students in US higher education. *Journal of Social Distress and Homelessness, 29*(1), 25–38.

Browning, M. H. E. M., Larson, L. R., Sharaievska, I., Rigolon, A., McAnirlin, O., Mullenbach, L., Cloutier, S., Vu, T. M., Thomsen, J., Reigner, N., Metcalf, E. C., D'Antonio, A., Helbich, M., Bratman, G. N., & Alvarez, H. O. (2021). Psychological impacts from COVID-19 among university students: Risk factors across seven states in the United States. *PLoS One, 16*(1), 1–27. https://doi.org/10.1371/journal.pone.0245327

Bureau, U. C. (2020). *Working moms bear brunt of home schooling while working during COVID-19.* https://www.census.gov/library/stories/2020/08/parents-juggle-work-and-child-care-during-pandemic.html

Buzzetto-Hollywood, N. (2021). Findings from an examination of a class purposed to teach the scientific method applied to the business discipline. *Issues in Informing Science & Information Technology, 18,* 161–172. a9h.

Chernozhukov, V., Kasahara, H., & Schrimpf, P. (2021). The association of opening K--12 schools with the spread of COVID-19 in the United States: County-level panel data analysis. *Proceedings of the National Academy of Sciences of the United States of America, 118*(42), 1–12. https://doi.org/10.1073/pnas.2103420118

Crawford, B. J., & Simon, M. S. (2021). Law faculty experiences teaching during the pandemic. *St. Louis University Law Journal, 65*(3), 455–470.

Crenshaw, K. W. (2017). *On intersectionality: Essential writings.* The New Press.

Cullen, R. (2001). Addressing the digital divide. *Online Information Review, 25*(5), 311–320. https://doi.org/10.1108/14684520110410517

Francom, G. M., Lee, S. J., & Pinkney, H. (2021). Technologies, challenges and needs of K-12 teachers in the transition to distance learning during the COVID-19 pandemic. *TechTrends: Linking Research & Practice to Improve Learning, 65*(4), 589–601. a9h.

Fry, R. (2022, June 14). Some gender disparities widened in the U.S. workforce during the pandemic. *Pew Research Center.* https://www.pewresearch.org/fact-tank/2022/01/14/some-gender-disparities-widened-in-the-u-s-workforce-during-the-pandemic/

Gupta, S., & Jawanda, M. (2020). The impacts of COVID-19 on children. *Acta Paediatrica, 109.* https://doi.org/10.1111/apa.15484

Gonzales, M. (2022, February 17). *Nearly 2 million fewer women in labor force.* SHRM. https://www.shrm.org/resourcesandtools/hr-topics/behavioral-competencies/global-and-cultural-effectiveness/pages/over-1-million-fewer-women-in-labor-force.aspx

Gorski, P. (2005). Education equity and the digital divide. *AACE Review (Formerly AACE Journal), 13*(1), 3–45.

Hallett, R. E., & Freas, A. (2018). Community college students' experiences with homelessness and housing insecurity. *Community College Journal of Research and Practice, 42*(10), 724–739.

Hall-Mills, S., Johnson, L., Gross, M., Latham, D., & Everhart, N. (2022). Providing telepractice in schools during a pandemic: The experiences and perspectives of speech-language pathologists. *Language, Speech & Hearing Services in Schools, 53*, 290–306. a9h.

Hash, P. M. (2021). Remote learning in school bands during the COVID-19 shutdown. *Journal of Research in Music Education, 68*(4), 381–397. a9h.

Haskett, M. E., Kotter-Grühn, D., & Majumder, S. (2020). Prevalence and correlates of food insecurity and homelessness among university students. *Journal of College Student Development, 61*(1), 109–114.

Huang, J. (2020). Successes and challenges: Online teaching and learning of chemistry in higher education in China in the time of COVID-19. *Journal of Chemical Education, 97*, 2810–2814. https://dx.doi.org/10.1021/acs.jchemed.0c00671

Jalongo, M. R. (2021). The effects of COVID-19 on early childhood education and care: Research and resources for children, families, teachers, and teacher educators. *Early Childhood Education Journal, 49*(5), 763–774. https://doi.org/10.1007/s10643-021-01208-y

Johnson, J., Daum, D., & Norris, J. (2021). I need help! Physical educators transition to distance learning during COVID-19. *Physical Educator, 78*(2), 119–137. https://doi.org/10.18666/tpe-2021-v78-i2-10866

Lanius, M., Jones, T. F., Kao, S., Lazarus, T., & Farrell, A. (2022). Unmotivated, depressed, anxious: Impact of the COVID-19 emergency transition to remote learning on undergraduates' Math Anxiety. *Journal of Humanistic Mathematics, 12*(1), 148–171. a9h.

Lederer, A. M., Hoban, M. T., Lipson, S. K., Zhou, S., & Eisenberg, D. (2021). More than inconvenienced: The unique needs of U.S. college students during the COVID-19 pandemic. *Health Education & Behavior, 48*(1), 14–19. https://doi.org/10.1177/1090198120969372

Luscombe, B. (2020). The rise of the "Carebnb". *TIME Magazine, 196*(16/17), 57–60.

McKenna, M., Soto-Boykin, X., Cheng, K., Haynes, E., Osorio, A., & Altshuler, J. (2021). Initial development of a national survey on remote learning in early childhood during COVID-19: Establishing content validity and reporting successes and barriers. *Early Childhood Education Journal, 49*(5), 815–827. https://doi.org/10.1007/s10643-021-01216-y

McQuate, S. (2020, April 14). How families can use technology to juggle childcare and remote life. *UW News.* https://www.washington.edu/news/2020/04/14/how-families-can-use-technology-to-juggle-childcare-and-remote-life/

Moldavan, A. M., Capraro, R. M., & Capraro, M. M. (2022). Navigating (and Disrupting) the digital divide: Urban teachers' perspectives on secondary mathematics instruction during COVID-19. *Urban Review, 54*(2), 277–302. a9h.

Mossa-Basha, M., Medverd, J., Linnau, K. F., Lynch, J. B., Wener, M. H., Kicska, G., Staiger, T., & Sahani, D. V. (2020). Policies and guidelines for COVID-19 preparedness: Experiences from the University of Washington. *Radiology, 296*(2), E26–E31.

Mustapha, I., Van, N. T., Shahverdi, M., Qureshi, M. I., & Khan, N. (2021). Effectiveness of digital technology in education during COVID-19 pandemic. *A Bibliometric Analysis, 136–154.* https://doi.org/10.3991/ijim.v15i08.20415

Panja, A., & Choudhury, S. M. (2022). Role of Science, technology and innovation for responding to Covid-19. *Asian Journal of Medical Sciences, 13*(3), 176–181. a9h.

Reich, J., Buttimer, C. J., Fang, A., Hillaire, G., Hirsch, K., Larke, L. R., Littenberg-Tobias, J., Moussapour, R. M., Napier, A., & Thompson, M. (2020). *Remote learning guidance from state education agencies during the COVID-19 pandemic: A first look.*

Richards, E., Quintana, C., Schnell, L., & Wong, A. (2021, March 21). A year after COVID-19 shut schools, students and teachers share what shook them – and what strengthened them. https://www.usatoday.com/in-depth/news/education/2021/03/21/covid-online-school-1-year-teachers-kids-share-powerful-quotes/4652348001/

Schafer, E. C., Dunn, A., & Lavi, A. (2021). Educational challenges during the pandemic for students who have hearing loss. *Language, Speech & Hearing Services in Schools, 52*(3), 889–898. a9h.

Simmons, D. (2020). Why COVID-19 is our equity check. *Educational Leadership, 77,* 51–53. [Special report]. http://www.ascd.org/publications/educational_leadership/summer20/vol77/num10/Why_COVID-19_Is_Our_Equity_Check.aspx

Slavin, R. E., & Storey, N. (2020). *The US Educational Response to the COVID-19 Pandemic* (SSRN Scholarly Paper No. 3652585). https://papers.ssrn.com/abstract=3652585

Son, C., Hegde, S., Smith, A., Wang, X., & Sasangohar, F. (2020). Effects of COVID-19 on college students' mental health in the United States: Interview survey study. *Journal of Medical Internet Research, 22*(9), e21279. https://doi.org/10.2196/21279

van Dijk, J. A. G. M. (2006). Digital divide research, achievements and shortcomings. *Poetics, 34*(4–5), 221–235. https://doi.org/10.1016/j.poetic.2006.05.004

Wang, X., Hegde, S., Son, C., Keller, B., Smith, A., & Sasangohar, F. (2020). Investigating mental health of US college students during the COVID-19 pandemic: Cross-sectional survey study. *Journal of Medical Internet Research, 22*(9), e22817. https://doi.org/10.2196/22817

Williams, P. (2020, April 8). *Delivery robots keep rolling during campus closure.* George Mason University News. https://content.sitemasonry.gmu.edu/news/2020-04/delivery-robots-keep-rolling-during-campus-closure

Winkle-Wagner, R. (2009). The perpetual homelessness of college experiences: Tensions between home and campus for African American women. *The Review of Higher Education, 33*(1), 1–36.

6

Access to Services and Resources

"This year has ushered in a new era of retail, and customers are asking for retailers to show up differently"

John Crecelius, Walmart (2020)

Access to services and resources is critical during extreme events. Several studies posited that the length and difficulty of recovery are often directly correlated with individual and household access to resources (Wisner, 2014; Riad, Norris, and Ruback, 1999; Cannon 1994). Resources have typically included access to finances, loved ones, communication, food, or spiritual guidance. Amid the pandemic, many of the resources needed to continue daily function (such as those offered by government agencies, social services, and nonprofit volunteer organizations) reduced their face-to-face interaction to minimize the risk of infection. The technological innovations developed during COVID remarkably allowed government agencies and social organizations to reach a wider proportion of the population. However, in some cases, technological innovations were inaccessible to the people most in need.

Though these new methods reached more people, it does not mean that all adopted the latest technology (device or software). When using new software or devices to connect with government agencies, some populations were warier about privacy and security concerns (see more in Chapter 9). Individual problems were with the use of their data for additional purposes or caution around the potential for surveillance (Madianou, 2020). Furthermore, technological innovations through public-private partnerships amid COVID were perceived as the start of a "digital" or "screen New Deal," as was signaled to some by the appointment of the former head of Google by former Governor Andrew Cuomo to "rethink New York City" post-pandemic (Madianou, 2020).

DOI: 10.1201/9781003319894-8

In this chapter, the innovative shifts to leverage various broadband wireless technologies during the pandemic are outlined based on how they were used; to minimize the spread in government buildings and ensure the continuity of government services, including for our justice system, law enforcement, and emergency management. Also included in this chapter are the innovations employed for the continuity of social services, such as food distribution, social work, and shelters.

As with many other sectors (e.g., education or public health guidance), state-level guidance varied. This likely increased the difficulty for individuals with disabilities or others with special needs. In fact, early in the pandemic there was an increase in the number of households that moved across state lines. In September of 2020, interstate moves increased by 32% from the previous year (United Van Lines, 2020). Comparing data on the top ten inbound and outbound household relocations during the first six months of the pandemic from UniGroup with the Johns Hopkins University Coronavirus Center data tracking the virus by state over time indicates the potential influence that the weekly infection rate, death rate, and infection rate had on interstate move decisions (see Table 6.1). Note that two states, Oregon and Masschusetts, appear on both top ten lists.

While physical health may have been a factor, access to services, resources, and loved ones also played a role in the decision-making process (Haslag & Weagley, 2022). In fact, a study by Haslag and Weagley (2022) showed that there was a significant decrease (13.5%) among households moving for job opportunities during COVID (as compared to pre-COVID numbers). However, moving for family and lifestyle showed a significant increase during COVID (Haslag & Weagley, 2022). In some states, services were difficult to access for individuals lacking technical prowess. For example, in Florida, teens created a nonprofit business to aid older adults in the use of new technologies, which became required (or highly desirable) during the pandemic (Susskind, 2020).

6.1 Mitigating the Virus

As essential businesses and services were required to commence amid social isolation and quarantine mandates, many were forced to adopt technologies to help mitigate the spread of the virus among workers,

Table 6.1   Comparison of Highest 7-Day Infection, Deaths, and Hospitalization Averages by State for the Top Ten Interstate Moves between March 2020 and August 2020

TOP TEN OUTBOUND STATES[a]	HIGHEST 7-DAY AVERAGES BETWEEN MARCH AND AUGUST 2020[b]	TOP TEN INBOUND STATES[a]	HIGHEST 7-DAY AVERAGES BETWEEN MARCH AND AUGUST 2020[b]
Washington D.C.	Cases = 194 Deaths= 12 Hospitalization = 520	Vermont	Cases = 41 Deaths = 2 Hospitalization = 53
New York	Cases = 10,843 Deaths = 1,014 Hospitalization = 13, 623	North Dakota	Cases = 77 Deaths = 2 Hospitalization = 76
Nevada	Cases = 1,155 Deaths = 15 Hospitalization = 1,261	Connecticut	Cases = 896 Deaths = 114 Hospitalization = 2,005
Oregon	Cases = 344 Deaths = 6 Hospitalization = 269	Montana	Cases = 129 Deaths = 1 Hospitalization = 86
Delaware	Cases = 211 Deaths = 11 Hospitalization = 342	Michigan	Cases = 1,670 Deaths = 146 Hospitalization = 3,727
California	Cases = 9,627 Deaths = 133 Hospitalization = 9,106	Arkansas	Cases = 817 Deaths = 10 Hospitalization = 1681
Minnesota	Cases = 706 Deaths = 25 Hospitalization = 805	Oregon	Cases = 344 Deaths = 6 Hospitalization = 269
Massachusetts	Cases = 2,226 Deaths = 189 Hospitalization = 4,292	Massachusetts	Cases = 2,226 Deaths = 189 Hospitalization = 4,292
Florida	Cases = 11,870 Deaths = 175 Hospitalization = 11,987	Ohio	Cases = 903 Deaths = 45 Hospitalization = 1959
Washington	Cases = 899 Deaths = 26 Hospitalization = 803	Utah	Cases = 670 Deaths = 5 Hospitalization = 292

[a] Data collected from UniGroup between March and August of 2020 https://www.unitedvanlines.com/newsroom/covid-moving-trends

[b] Data collected from Johns Hopkins University Coronavirus Resource Center https://coronavirus.jhu.edu/region

clients, and constituents. Forehead thermometer checks, thermal cameras, and other means for remote thermal detection were used in jails, ports of entry (such as airports), government buildings (including the White House), as well as businesses, hospitals, and grocery stores (Van Natta et al., 2020).

Some state governments developed and released contact tracing and proof of vaccination mobile applications to help minimize the spread of the virus (Hendl et al., 2020; Sato, 2020; Van Ness, 2021; Yuan et al., 2022). While globally, some countries introduced these measures with national guidance. A handful of state governments in the U.S. implemented mobile apps for COVID; however, few worked across jurisdictions. Chapter 7 provides information related to the use of technology in healthcare, while Chapter 8 provides more detail on the mobile applications introduced during the pandemic. In conjunction with mobile apps, some governments employed drones and land-based robots to help with social distancing (BBC News, 2020; Sathyamoorthy et al., 2021).

6.2 Emergency Management

Even though there was the global response, recovery, and mitigation of the coronavirus, other disasters also occurred. In 2020 alone, there were 22 major disaster events from severe storms, drought, wildfire, and hurricanes. These disasters impacted the U.S., for a total of $95 billion in damages, not counting the pandemic (Smith, 2021). All of which required a comprehensive, cohesive, and coordinated emergency management response. As such there were several innovative strategies developed, such as the change in location for strategic planning: the emergency operations center (EOC) moved online. The EOC, used as a coordination and planning hub during disasters, was often thought of as a *physical* location where critical stakeholders typically sit together to rapidly make decisions and analyze real-time information about the current incident. However, the EOC in many locations moved virtually, for some, and allowed stakeholders to be readily available and share information and minimize risk of infectious disease (Holdeman, 2022). Other innovative strategies included non-congregated sheltering, outdoor evacuation points, spray grounds, automatic person counters for crowd management, software for emergency management resources (FEMA, 2020b; Indiana University

News, 2020; Rinde, 2020). These tools helped emergency management professionals continue preparedness and response efforts for other ongoing hazards such as wildfires, hurricanes, and heat waves amid the pandemic.

6.3 Law Enforcement

In some locations, COVID-related data was shared with police departments to assist in mitigation efforts (Kruesi, 2021; Molldrem et al., 2021; Protecting Minnesota's First Responders By Directing the Commissioner of Health to Share Information with the Department of Public Safety, 911 Dispatchers, and First Responders, 2020). The potential for increased fear and discriminatory tactics based on COVID-related public health data was noted by several academics in disciplines such as social sciences, criminal justice, and public health. Several states shared some level of data with law enforcement such as who received a COVID test. In fact, 35 states provided addresses of people who tested positive with law enforcement, and ten of those states also shared the names (Gomez-Barrero et al., 2022; Guariglia, 2020). In Tennessee, bipartisan lawmakers were significantly upset and some cited that this level of data sharing would increase mistrust among community, which would lead to a reduction in individuals willing to get tested (Kruesi, 2021). In other areas there was concern that the information would be shared with immigration officials, who continued deportations even though doing so may have contributed to spread of the virus (Cénat, 2020; Garcini et al., 2020; Ross et al., 2021).

Facial recognition, geographic tracking, and thermal imaging cameras were used to collect data for both public health and law enforcement (Guariglia, 2020). In some cases, the mitigation efforts for COVID hindered the use of technology by law enforcement. Masks prohibited effective use of facial recognition software, and hand sanitizer, used as a disinfectant, had a side effect of drying hands, which reduces the amount of moisture needed for some fingerprint analyses (Gomez-Barrero et al., 2022).

6.4 Driving Licensure

During the pandemic, several government services were quickly updated and provided through an online environment. Motor vehicle, matrimonial, and even legal services were conducted in part online or without in-person interaction. The majority of state departments of motor vehicles (DMV) adapted their road tests for the pandemic (31 states), all adopted at least one policy, and 49 states allowed for renewal extensions (Feiss et al., 2021). Many states allowed written exams to be taken online and at home. However, states with road tests issued a waiver, outsourced the test to a driving school, or were conducted in-person with extra health-related precautions. For example, Georgia issued drivers licenses to nearly 20,000 teens without requiring a road test to address backlog issues (Feiss et al., 2021; Taylor, 2020). In Montana and Colorado renewals were conducted online or by mail in, however, in Arkansas, drivers had to process everything in person, nothing was available online (Feiss et al., 2021). Only eight state DMVs had precautions outlined that were specific to older adults. Delaware also specified hours for older adults and other vulnerable populations (Feiss et al., 2021).

Additionally, the empty roads due to the lockdowns contributed to riskier behavior among the few on the road. Speed driving increased by 43% during normal rush hour times in Virginia, without the rush hour traffic (Young, 2022). Crash deaths increased 4% in 2020. According to the National Highway Traffic Administration (NHTSA) these increased deaths were likely due to speeding, intoxication, or lack of a seatbelt (Young, 2022). These patterns held steady or increased in 2021.

6.5 Legal Matters

Legal matters, including divorces, were handled in part online, as well (Baldwin et al., 2020). In April 2020, the judicial conference requested 36.6 million to assist with the adjustments needed to maintain the continuity of operations, through, among other things, the expanded use of technology (Hershkoff & Miller, 2020). However, this request was denied, but the lack of funds did not prohibit the transition to technology-facilitated legal arguments. In Texas, over 1,800 hearings were conducted by judges, virtually (Wienrich et al., 2022). Even the Supreme Court of the United States and state supreme courts held hearings and arguments virtually (Baldwin et al., 2020).

Court hearings and cases conducted via video conferencing software began to present various advantages and challenges. The use of such technology increased the accessibility and likelihood of fair and impartial trials. Furthermore, the use of technology may have helped to speed up the process of our lagging judicial system (Clare, 2021; Early & Hernandez, 2021; Sieck et al., 2021; Wienrich et al., 2022). Some researchers pointed out that the use of video conferencing posed concerns due to the difference in communication styles virtually vs. in-person (causing virtual fatigue or "Zoom fatigue"), increased strain due to learning the technology, and varied data protections of third-party solutions, such as Zoom and Microsoft Teams (Wienrich et al., 2022). Not to mention the technical challenges posed by providing off-site access to personnel records and hosting attorney/climate privileged meetings, when conducting all aspects of our judicial system online. These challenges may have affected the protection of rights and full participation (Hershkoff & Miller, 2020; Wienrich et al., 2022). To protect rights and make proceedings accessible, many courts began to stream online, in real time (Baldwin et al., 2020). But it did not address issues of fairness when one's first language is not English, or with individuals who were blind, had low vision, or were deaf (Hershkoff & Miller, 2020).

On top of this, the legal matters increased during the pandemic, as some suggested there were "twin pandemics," one due to COVID and the other due to increased racism (Hershkoff & Miller, 2020). There were disproportionate racist and violent attacks targeted to racial and ethnic minorities facilitated through technology, primarily toward Black and Asian American populations (Bailey et al., 2021; Ruiz et al., 2020; Yang et al., 2020).

6.6 Pandemic Matrimonies

The pandemic affected marriages as well. Not only were marriage certificates obtained via the internet, in some states the ceremonies were conducted virtually (Dubois et al., 2022). There was an estimated 12% decline in marriages during 2020, though the declines varied by state (Westrick-Payne & Wendy Manning, 2022), where, for example, Texas and Montana recorded an increase in marriages.

However, Montana's double proxy policy for wedding ceremonies may have contributed to the increase (Westrick-Payne & Wendy Manning, 2022). Double proxy marriages allowed for both people elsewhere in the country while getting married.

Marriage ceremonies changed amid the pandemic, some saying "I do" with virtual attendees and others opting for smaller more intimate weddings. The culture of having elaborate weddings may have changed, as well, where people were once spending over $30,000 for their big day to under $1,000, amid the pandemic, opting for an online or civil ceremony at a courthouse (Aviles, 2020; Gachman, 2021). Many states legalized online weddings, including New York (Crowley, 2020). In an online wedding, the officiant was also virtual. However, the executive order from Governor Cuomo was no longer viable after the state of emergency ended. After which, the officiant and couple must be physically present in the same space, making the ceremony in-person, but couples could still have the ceremony live streamed for virtual attendees.

There were fewer legal divorces in 2020, with larger declines in Louisiana and Maryland (Westrick-Payne & Wendy Manning, 2022). However, overall, the pandemic may have led to an increase in breakups among both married and unmarried couples, some forced to quarantine together. In fact, there is some evidence to suggest that discussions related to science of the COVID reality, response, impacts, and vaccination may have contributed to couples reaching a breaking point, especially true for those married longer (Ellyatt, 2022; Goldberg et al., 2021; Maher, 2021; Westrick-Payne & Wendy Manning, 2022).

6.7 Personal Activities

The collective move online challenged individual access to daily activities. Where once people had the option to participate in activities face-to-face, amid the pandemic, the choice was often to either pivot online or go without. The access issues were related to a myriad of concerns; determining if the activity could be performed the same way online, the website design, the mobile app, the digital literacy of the user, or knowledge (and adoption) of the new software or hardware that may be required.

Social isolation for many became nearly unbearable, and mental health issues soared. Older adults and children are often among the most vulnerable due to social isolation-induced psychological distress (Drouin et al., 2020; Loades et al., 2020; Sepúlveda-Loyola et al., 2020). In some cases, increased use of technology, primarily social media, among these groups reduced distress caused by the quarantine (Cosco et al., 2021; Eghtesadi, 2020; Kasar & Karaman, 2021; Marston et al., 2020). Among individuals 70 and older, research suggested that the use of social media to maintain social connections may have helped. In contrast, the impact on the use of video-based software among older adults was not as clear (Kasar & Karaman, 2021). In another study, the use of pet robots was explored as a means to reduce the impacts of social isolation (Van Orden et al., 2022). Additionally, both children and their parents increased their use of technology during the isolation to quell the anxiety (Drouin et al., 2020). Chapter 7 discusses more information about mental health challenges.

In response to anxiety and distress, people looked for ways to continue other daily activities to be social and physical. Some picked up new hobbies and recreational activities. The fishing industry, as a COVID-19 safe activity, rose significantly during the pandemic (Midway et al., 2021). Cooking became a pastime that increased during the pandemic. However, supply chain issues threatened the ability to rely on the availability of healthy food. As such, other COVID-19 safe hobbies increased as well, namely gardening (Wilkins, 2020).

The purchase of groceries online increased from 3–4% to 10–15% over the pandemic. The purchase of groceries through online vendors and websites rose as the cases of infection rose (Grashuis et al., 2020). Similarly, the use of third-party apps for prepared food delivery from restaurants increased (Dubois et al., 2022); although, the use of mobile applications to purchase groceries proved to be challenging for some older adults (Xie et al., 2020). As such, volunteer matching programs and nonprofit groups emerged across the country to assist older adults (Du Sault, 2020; Susskind, 2020). These programs connected older adults to lower-risk individuals who could pick up groceries, prescriptions, and event assist with the use of broadband wireless technologies for telehealth, socialization, and access to government services.

Other people flocked to technology to aid in the continuity of leisure activities; even sexual activity was maintained with the assistance of technology (Eleuteri & Terzitta, 2021). Many innovative technologies were quickly developed, apps and devices, to assist fitness buffs in at-home workouts during the pandemic (Dubois et al., 2022; Godefroy, 2020). Social media influencers used their pages to promote exercises that could be done at home, and fitness centers offered online fitness sessions to maintain their customer base (Godefroy, 2020; Kim et al., 2022). Fitness devices were frequently part of online purchases (Chiu et al., 2022). The search for fitness apps online increased by 46% in one quarter during the pandemic (Clark & Lupton, 2021).

Impulse buyers were challenged by the general increase in online shopping, which led to hedonistic buying (Chiu et al., 2022; Clark & Lupton, 2021). There is some evidence to suggest that impulse buying during the pandemic was in part driven by fear, and more significantly so for lower-income populations (Chiu et al., 2022). Though lower-income populations may have an impulse to buy, amid increased fear during COVID, little is known about their use of these purchases (Chiu et al., 2022). Whereas at least one study in Australia was able to determine the extent to which individuals rearranged their living spaces due to technology to accommodate an atmosphere for taking care of the mind, body, and soul (Clark & Lupton, 2021).

6.8 Religious Activities

Pre-pandemic, places of worship were a refuge for replenishing the soul. But, during the pandemic, religious traditions, ceremonies, and celebrations were also affected. In the U.S., lockdown mandates and guidance began just at the start of many annual religious events during the spring; Passover for Jewish populations, Easter for Christians, and Ramadan (and the Hajj) for Muslim populations (Campbell, 2020; Parish, 2020). As such, there were several adaptations; virtual services became more of a norm, as parishioners convened over videoconferencing software or live streaming (Campbell, 2020; Parish, 2020; Wiederhold, 2020). With regard to religious holidays, many Easter services were conducted at the drive-in theater for safety (Wiederhold, 2020). One of the most disruptive of all, the Hajj pilgrimage was canceled (Campbell, 2020). Furthermore, even funerals were conducted using internet-based technology (Burrell & Selman, 2022; Pitsillides & Wallace, 2021). As the pandemic death toll climbed so did the need for social distant funeral services. The funeral industry was also forced online; live streaming services, drive by wakes, gravesite burials on AM/FM radio (Wells, 2020).

Houses of worship able to pivot to online methods for the delivery of services also encountered challenges. However, there was evidence that online services opened to a wider audience (Campbell, 2020). Members became more actively engaged, and marginalized populations were able to bond together online. For example, African American Muslims held and attended religious discussions online (Campbell, 2020). However, smaller churches struggled to keep their parishioners and maintain funding (Boorstein, 2020). COVID-19 may have pushed the reinvention of religious services, but not just during the pandemic. Questions circulate about the future of religious services and the relationship between religion and online technology (Parish, 2020).

Religious organizations were not only innovative in the delivery of worship services, but they were also instrumental in the delivery of mission services to assist during the pandemic globally (Derose & Mata, 2020). In truth, faith-based organizations have regularly been instrumental in response and recovery efforts following disasters (Ngin et al., 2020; Phillips & Jenkins, 2010; Rivera & Nickels, 2014; Sakai, 2012; Stajura et al., 2012). In the U.S., Samaritan's purse created a 68-bed emergency hospital in NY Central Park for critical COVID patients (USAID, 2020), and the State Department commended religious-based organizations for their efforts to reduce vaccination hesitancy and in the fight against human rights injustices amid the pandemic (US Department of State, 2021). However, it is important to note that some religious leaders were the source of the anti-vax movements in the U.S. and abroad (Govender, 2022; Hals, 2021).

6.9 Human and Social Services

Nonprofits lost a sizable percentage of their workforce during the pandemic (both salaried and volunteer employees), though most experienced an increase in demand (FEMA, 2020a). School-based and culture-related organizations had to contend with 100% closure

(FEMA, 2020a). Several providers shifted to online delivery of services where applicable; this was especially true in California (Holliday et al., 2020). However, service providers faced several barriers with funding, lack of technology access among clients, and workforce decreases, among others (Holliday et al., 2020).

But there were positive changes; COVID forced public health, healthcare and social services to find unique means of working together (Landers et al., 2020). A number of funding opportunities and pilot policies allowed for shared mission, goals, and data to promote healthy well-being for marginalized communities (Landers et al., 2020). However, community-based social services were woefully understaffed or significantly restricted as a non-essential service (Petchel, 2020). Community-based homeless and domestic violence organizations were hampered by the COVID-19 response and resorted to relying on technology (Altheimer et al., 2020; Fedorowicz et al., 2020). And there were challenges with obtaining appropriate technologies or devices for public facing workers, digital literacy, and having the proper upgrades to use newer technology.

The ethical practice of social work and social justice may have also been challenged by technology, globally. As many in these professions rely on the ability to foster trust and openness in the relationships with their clients, the required distance and use of a virtual environment increased the difficulty of making meaningful connections (Banks et al., 2020). Some clients worried about their privacy. Furthermore, the virtual experience impeded their ability to make proper assessments, for home visits or of domestic abuse.

For those working with sexual minorities, such as nonprofit advocacy groups, there was an increase in discrimination and hate (particularly online), leaving members of the LGBTQ community at a heightened vulnerability. Many were unwilling to partake of some services such as meal delivery, homeless shelters, or child services – even if facilitated online (Farkas & Romaniuk, 2020). Another indication of the impact of the "twin pandemics."

Disability-related organizations found that the use of technology allowed them to reinvent the way in which services were offered. Technology allowed clients to connect with loved ones (especially those with mobility disabilities). Some organizations, however, encountered challenges with the use of technology for the continuation of operations (Hughes et al., 2022). For example, the use of video conferencing was not necessarily an appropriate technology due to a lack of digital literacy among the clients.

6.10 Summary

Access to services and resources changed drastically during the pandemic. Services provided by government agencies, private businesses, and nonprofit organizations all continued due to internal policies that leveraged broadband wireless-based information and communications technologies. From the way mitigation efforts, monitored and legal arguments were held, government agencies encountered new benefits and challenges primarily because of public perception, ethical concerns, and ease of use. As stress and isolation increased during the pandemic, private businesses offered a myriad of activities and means to socialize using various technologies. Nonprofit organizations, including faith-based houses of worship, were also affected by the pandemic, having to shift to virtual methods of delivering services and fostering community. The digital divide, digital literacy, privacy concerns, and issues of digital equity challenged wide support of some innovative solutions. Furthermore, the second of the twin pandemics – increased racism – created barriers to full participation for some, and increased concern about safety for others.

References

Altheimer, I., Duda-Banwar, J., & Schreck, C. J. (2020). The impact of Covid-19 on community-based violence interventions. *American Journal of Criminal Justice*, *45*(4), 810–819. https://doi.org/10.1007/s12103-020-09547-z

Aviles, G. (2020). How coronavirus could change wedding culture—Even after the pandemic ends. *NBC News*. https://www.nbcnews.com/pop-culture/pop-culture-news/how-coronavirus-could-change-wedding-culture-even-after-pandemic-ends-n1185506

Bailey, J., Flynn, A., & Henry, N. (2021). Pandemics and systemic discrimination: Technology-facilitated violence and abuse in an era of COVID-19 and antiracist protest. In J. Bailey, A. Flynn, & N. Henry (Eds.), *The emerald international handbook of technology-facilitated violence and abuse* (pp. 787–797). Emerald Publishing Limited. https://doi.org/10.1108/978-1-83982-848-520211057

Baldwin, J. M., Eassey, J. M., & Brooke, E. J. (2020). Court operations during the COVID-19 Pandemic. *American Journal of Criminal Justice*, *45*(4), 743–758. https://doi.org/10.1007/s12103-020-09553-1

Banks, S., Cai, T., de Jonge, E., Shears, J., Shum, M., Sobočan, A. M., Strom, K., Truell, R., Úriz, M. J., & Weinberg, M. (2020). Practising ethically during COVID-19: Social work challenges and responses. *International Social Work*, *63*(5), 569–583. https://doi.org/10.1177/0020872820949614

BBC News. (2020, May 11). *Coronavirus: Robot dog enforces social distancing in Singapore park—BBC News*. https://www.bbc.com/news/av/technology-52619568

Boorstein, M. (2020, April 24). Church donations have plunged because of the coronavirus. Some churches won't survive. *Washington Post*. https://www.washingtonpost.com/religion/2020/04/24/church-budgets-coronavirus-debt/

Burrell, A., & Selman, L. E. (2022). How do funeral practices impact bereaved relatives' mental health, grief and bereavement? A mixed methods review with implications for COVID-19. *OMEGA - Journal of Death and Dying*, *85*(2), 345–383. https://doi.org/10.1177/0030222820941296

Campbell, H. (2020). *Religion in quarantine: The future of religion in a post-pandemic world*. https://oaktrust.library.tamu.edu/bitstream/handle/1969.1/188004/Religion%20in%20Quarantine-PDF-eBook-final-2020.pdf?sequence=4

Cannon, T. (1994). Vulnerability analysis and the explanation of 'natural' disasters. *Disasters, Development and Environment*, *1*, 13–30.

Cénat, J. M. (2020). US deportation policies in the time of COVID-19: A public health threat to the Americas. *Public Health*, *185*, 4–5. https://doi.org/10.1016/j.puhe.2020.05.017

Chiu, W., (Grace) Oh, G.-E., & Cho, H. (2022). Impact of COVID-19 on consumers' impulse buying behavior of fitness products: A moderated mediation model. *Journal of Consumer Behaviour*, *21*(2), 245–258. https://doi.org/10.1002/cb.1998

Clare, C. A. (2021). Telehealth and the digital divide as a social determinant of health during the COVID-19 pandemic. *Network Modeling Analysis in Health Informatics and Bioinformatics*, *10*(1), 26. https://doi.org/10.1007/s13721-021-00300-y

Clark, M., & Lupton, D. (2021). Pandemic fitness assemblages: The socio-materialities and affective dimensions of exercising at home during the COVID-19 crisis. *Convergence*, *27*(5), 1222–1237. https://doi.org/10.1177/13548565211042460

Cosco, T. D., Fortuna, K., Wister, A., Riadi, I., Wagner, K., & Sixsmith, A. (2021). COVID-19, social isolation, and mental health among older adults: A digital catch-22. *Journal of Medical Internet Research*, *23*(5), e21864. https://doi.org/10.2196/21864

Crowley, J. (2020, April 30). Getting married online is now legal in New York. *Newsweek*. https://www.newsweek.com/project-cupid-new-york-coronavirus-weddings-online-marriage-license-1501252

Derose, K. P., & Mata, M. (2020, April 16). *The Role of Faith-Based Organiza_tions During the Pandemic.* https://www.rand.org/blog/2020/04/the-important-role-of-faith-based-organizations-in.html

Drouin, M., McDaniel, B. T., Pater, J., & Toscos, T. (2020). How parents and their children used social media and technology at the beginning of the COVID-19 pandemic and associations with anxiety. *Cyberpsychology, Behavior, and Social Networking, 23*(11), 727–736.

Du Sault, Laurence. (2020, July 21). The CA seniors left behind by a telehealth tech divide. Patch. https://patch.com/california/across-ca/coronavirus-bay-area-seniors-who-are-left-behind-telehealth-tech-divide

Dubois, E., Yuan, X., Bennett Gayle, D., Khurana, P., Knight, T., Laforce, S., Turetsky, D., & Wild, D. (2022). Socially vulnerable populations adoption of technology to address lifestyle changes amid COVID-19 in the US. *Data and Information Management, 6*(2), 100001–100001. https://doi.org/10.1016/j.dim.2022.100001

Early, J., & Hernandez, A. (2021). Digital disenfranchisement and COVID-19: Broadband internet access as a social determinant of health. *Health Promotion Practice, 22*(5), 605–610. https://doi.org/10.1177/15248399211014490

Eghtesadi, M. (2020). Breaking social isolation amidst COVID-19: A viewpoint on improving access to technology in long-term care facilities. *Journal of the American Geriatrics Society, 68*(5), 949.

Eleuteri, S., & Terzitta, G. (2021). Sexuality during the COVID-19 pandemic: The importance of Internet. *Sexologies, 30*(1), e55–e60. https://doi.org/10.1016/j.sexol.2020.12.008

Ellyatt, H. (2022, January 21). Arguing with your partner over Covid? You're not alone, with the pandemic straining many relationships. *CNBC.* https://www.cnbc.com/2022/01/21/covid-has-put-pressures-and-strains-on-relationships.html

Farkas, K. J., & Romaniuk, J. R. (2020). Social work, ethics and vulnerable groups in the time of coronavirus and Covid-19. *Society Register, 4*(2), 67–82.

Fedorowicz, M., Arena, O., & Burrowes, K. (2020). *Community engagement during the COVID-19 pandemic and beyond a guide for community-based organizations.* Urban Institute. https://drum.lib.umd.edu/bitstream/handle/1903/26915/community-engagement-during-the-covid-19-pandemic-and-beyond.pdf?sequence=1

Feiss, R., Hautmann, A., Asa, N., Hamann, C., Peek-Asa, C., & Yang, J. (2021). Balancing safety on the road with risk from COVID-19: A content analysis of policy adaptations by divisions of motor vehicles. *Accident Analysis & Prevention, 162*, 106400. https://doi.org/10.1016/j.aap.2021.106400

FEMA. (2020a). COVID-19's impact on the human and social services sector. (p. 20). https://www.fema.gov/sites/default/files/2020-11/fema_covid-19-impact-human-social-services-sector_best-practice_11-16-20.pdf

FEMA. (2020b, May 31). Coronavirus (COVID-19) pandemic: Non-congregate sheltering | FEMA.gov. FEMA. https://www.fema.gov/news-release/20200722/coronavirus-covid-19-pandemic-non-congregate-sheltering

Gachman, D. (2021, September 16). Are Zoom weddings virtually over? *The New York Times*. https://www.nytimes.com/2021/09/16/style/virtual-weddings-over.html

Garcini, L. M., Mercado, A., Domenech Rodríguez, M. M., & Paris, M. (2020). A tale of two crises: The compounded effect of COVID-19 and anti-immigration policy in the United States. *Psychological Trauma : Theory, Research, Practice and Policy*, *12*(Suppl 1), S230–S232. https://doi.org/10.1037/tra0000775

Godefroy, J. (2020). Recommending physical activity during the COVID-19 health crisis. Fitness influencers on Instagram. *Frontiers in Sports and Active Living*, *2*. https://www.frontiersin.org/articles/10.3389/fspor.2020.589813

Goldberg, A. E., Allen, K. R., & Smith, J. Z. (2021). Divorced and separated parents during the COVID-19 pandemic. *Family Process*, *60*(3), 866–887. https://doi.org/10.1111/famp.12693

Gomez-Barrero, M., Drozdowski, P., Rathgeb, C., Patino, J., Todisco, M., Nautsch, A., Damer, N., Priesnitz, J., Evans, N., & Busch, C. (2022). Biometrics in the era of COVID-19: Challenges and opportunities. *IEEE Transactions on Technology and Society*, *1–1*. https://doi.org/10.1109/TTS.2022.3203571

Govender, S. (2022, July 11). *Some religious leaders "have fuelled" South Africans' hesitancy to take Covid-19 vaccines*. https://www.timeslive.co.za/news/south-africa/2022-06-11-some-religious-leaders-have-fuelled-south-africans-hesitancy-to-take-covid-19-vaccines/

Grashuis, J., Skevas, T., & Segovia, M. S. (2020). Grocery shopping preferences during the COVID-19 pandemic. *Sustainability*, *12*(13), 5369.

Guariglia, M. (2020, April 15). *Telling police where people with COVID-19 live erodes public health*. Electronic Frontier Foundation. https://www.eff.org/deeplinks/2020/04/telling-police-where-people-covid-19-live-erodes-public-health

Hals, T. (2021, October 14). U.S. pastors, advocacy groups mobilize against COVID-19 vaccine mandates | Reuters. *Reuters*. https://www.reuters.com/world/us/us-pastors-advocacy-groups-mobilize-against-covid-19-vaccine-mandates-2021-10-14/

Haslag, P. H., & Weagley, D. (2022). From LA to Boise: How migration has changed during the COVID-19 pandemic. *Available at SSRN 3808326*.

Hendl, T., Chung, R., & Wild, V. (2020). Pandemic surveillance and racialized subpopulations: Mitigating vulnerabilities in COVID-19 apps. *Journal of Bioethical Inquiry*, *17*(4), 829–834. https://doi.org/10.1007/s11673-020-10034-7

Hershkoff, H., & Miller, A. R. (2020). Courts and civil justice in the time of COVID: Emerging trends and questions to ask. *New York University Journal of Legislation and Public Policy*, *23*(2), 321–424.

Holdeman, E. (2022, February 1). The Virtual EOC. *GovTech*. https://www.govtech.com/disaster-zone/the-virtual-eoc

Holliday, S. B., Hunter, S. B., Dopp, A. R., Chamberlin, M., & Iguchi, M. Y. (2020). *Exploring the impact of COVID-19 on social services for vulnerable populations in Los Angeles: Lessons learned from community providers.* RAND Corporation. https://www.rand.org/pubs/research_reports/RRA431-1. html

Hughes, M. C., Gray, J. A., & Kim, J. (2022). The perspective of administrators of intellectual disability organizations on the COVID-19 pandemic. *Journal of Intellectual Disabilities.* https://doi.org/10.1177/17446295211062400

Indiana University News. (2020, June 22). Free, public dashboard helps emergency managers share critical COVID-19 information. *Indiana University Information Technology News & Events.* https://itnews.iu.edu/ articles/2020/Free-public-dashboard-helps-emergency-managers-share-critical-COVID-19-information-.php#:~:text=Free%2C%20public%20 dashboard%20helps%20emergency,police%2C%20and%20health%20 and%20medical

Kasar, K. S., & Karaman, E. (2021). Life in lockdown: Social isolation, loneliness and quality of life in the elderly during the COVID-19 pandemic: A scoping review. *Geriatric Nursing, 42*(5), 1222–1229.

Kim, H.-M., Kim, M., & Cho, I. (2022). Home-based workouts in the era of COVID-19 pandemic: The influence of Fitness YouTubers' attributes on intentions to exercise. *Internet Research, ahead-of-print* (ahead-of-print). https://doi.org/10.1108/INTR-03-2021-0179

Kruesi, K. (2021, April 20). COVID-19 data sharing with law enforcement sparks concern. *AP NEWS.* https://apnews.com/article/nv-state-wire-nd-state-wire-co-state-wire-nh-state-wire-public-health-ab4cbfb5575671 c5630c2442bc3ca75e

Landers, G. M., Minyard, K. J., Lanford, D., & Heishman, H. (2020). A theory of change for aligning health care, public health, and social services in the time of COVID-19. In *American Journal of Public Health, 110*(S2), S178–S180). American Public Health Association.

Loades, M. E., Chatburn, E., Higson-Sweeney, N., Reynolds, S., Shafran, R., Brigden, A., Linney, C., McManus, M. N., Borwick, C., & Crawley, E. (2020). Rapid systematic review: The impact of social isolation and loneliness on the mental health of children and adolescents in the context of COVID-19. *Journal of the American Academy of Child & Adolescent Psychiatry, 59*(11), 1218–1239.e3. https://doi.org/10.1016/j. jaac.2020.05.009

Madianou, M. (2020). A second-order disaster? Digital technologies during the COVID-19 pandemic—Mirca Madianou, 2020. *Social Media and Society.* https://journals.sagepub.com/doi/full/10.1177/2056305120948168

Maher, K. (2021). *From locking down to lawyering up: COVID-19 and the later life divorce trend.* https://www.newyorklife.com/newsroom/seniors-gray-divorce

Marston, H. R., Musselwhite, C., & Hadley, R. A. (2020). COVID-19 vs social isolation: The impact technology can have on communities, social connections and citizens. *The British Society of Gerontology.*

Midway, S. R., Lynch, A. J., Peoples, B. K., Dance, M., & Caffey, R. (2021). COVID-19 influences on US recreational angler behavior. *PLoS One*, *16*(8), e0254652. https://doi.org/10.1371/journal.pone.0254652

Molldrem, S., Hussain, M. I., & McClelland, A. (2021). Alternatives to sharing COVID-19 data with law enforcement: Recommendations for stakeholders. *Health Policy*, *125*(2), 135–140. https://doi.org/10.1016/j.healthpol.2020.10.015

Ngin, C., Grayman, J. H., Neef, A., & Sanunsilp, N. (2020). The role of faith-based institutions in urban disaster risk reduction for immigrant communities. *Natural Hazards*, *103*(1), 299–316.

Parish, H. (2020). The absence of presence and the presence of absence: Social distancing, sacraments, and the virtual religious community during the COVID-19 pandemic. *Religions*, *11*(6), 276.

Petchel, S. (2020). COVID-19 makes funding for health and social services integration even more crucial. *Health Affairs Blog*. https://www.healthaffairs.org/do/10.1377/forefront.20200413.886531/full/

Phillips, B., & Jenkins, P. (2010). *The roles of faith-based organizations after Hurricane Katrina*.

Pitsillides, S., & Wallace, J. (2021). *Physically distant but socially connected: Streaming funerals, memorials and ritual design during COVID-19* (pp. 60–76). https://doi.org/10.4324/9781003125990-4-6

Protecting Minnesota's First Responders By Directing the Commissioner of Health to Share Information with the Department of Public Safety, 911 Dispatchers, and First Responders, no. Emergency Executive Order 20-34 (2020). https://www.leg.mn.gov/archive/execorders/20-34.pdf

Riad, J. K., Norris, F. H., & Ruback, R. B. (1999). Predicting evacuation in two major disasters: Risk perception, social influence, and access to resources 1. *Journal of Applied Social Psychology*, *29*(5), 918–934.

Rinde, M. (2020, July 7). Philadelphia opens spraygrounds, officials say they're safe for kids. *WHYY*. https://whyy.org/articles/spraygrounds-a-relatively-safe-way-to-cool-off-experts-say/

Rivera, J. D., & Nickels, A. E. (2014). Social capital, community resilience, and faith-based organizations in disaster recovery: A case study of Mary Queen of Vietnam Catholic Church. *Risk, Hazards & Crisis in Public Policy*, *5*(2), 178–211.

Ross, H. M., Desiderio, S., St. Mars, T., & Rangel, P. (2021). US immigration policies pose threat to health security during COVID-19 pandemic. *Health Security*, *19*(S1), S-83. https://doi.org/10.1089/hs.2021.0039

Ruiz, N. G., Horowitz, J. M., & Tamir, C. (2020, July 1). Many black and Asian Americans say they have experienced discrimination amid the COVID-19 outbreak. *Pew Research Center's Social & Demographic Trends Project*. https://www.pewresearch.org/social-trends/2020/07/01/many-black-and-asian-americans-say-they-have-experienced-discrimination-amid-the-covid-19-outbreak/

Sakai, M. (2012). Building a partnership for social service delivery in Indonesia: State and faith-based organisations. *Australian Journal of Social Issues*, *47*(3), 373–388.

Sathyamoorthy, A. J., Patel, U., Paul, M., Savle, Y., & Manocha, D. (2021). COVID surveillance robot: Monitoring social distancing constraints in indoor scenarios. *PLoS One, 16*(12), e0259713. https://doi.org/10.1371/journal.pone.0259713

Sato, M. (2020). Contact tracing apps now cover nearly half of America. It's not too late to use one. *MIT Technology Review*. https://www.technologyreview.com/2020/12/14/1014426/covid-california-contact-tracing-app-america-states/

Sepúlveda-Loyola, W., Rodríguez-Sánchez, I., Pérez-Rodríguez, P., Ganz, F., Torralba, R., Oliveira, D. V., & Rodríguez-Mañas, L. (2020). Impact of social isolation due to COVID-19 on health in older people: Mental and physical effects and recommendations. *The Journal of Nutrition, Health & Aging, 24*(9), 938–947. https://doi.org/10.1007/s12603-020-1500-7

Sieck, C. J., Sheon, A., Ancker, J. S., Castek, J., Callahan, B., & Siefer, A. (2021). Digital inclusion as a social determinant of health. *Npj Digital Medicine, 4*(1), Article 1. https://doi.org/10.1038/s41746-021-00413-8

Smith, A. (2021). *2020 U.S. billion-dollar weather and climate disasters in historical context*. NOAA Climate.gov. http://www.climate.gov/disasters2020

Stajura, M., Glik, D., Eisenman, D., Prelip, M., Martel, A., & Sammartinova, J. (2012). Perspectives of community-and faith-based organizations about partnering with local health departments for disasters. *International Journal of Environmental Research and Public Health, 9*(7), 2293–2311.

Susskind, S. (2020, December 31). *Palm Beach County teen helps seniors with technology during COVID-19 pandemic*. WPTV. https://www.wptv.com/news/region-c-palm-beach-county/riviera-beach/palm-beach-county-teen-helps-seniors-with-technology-during-covid-19-pandemic

Taylor, D. B. (2020, May 7). Nearly 20,000 Georgia teens are issued driver's licenses without a road test. *The New York Times*. https://www.nytimes.com/2020/05/07/us/georgia-teen-driving-test-coronavirus.html

United Van Lines (2020, October 6). COVID-19 moving trends and data insights. https://www.unitedvanlines.com/newsroom/covid-moving-trends

US Department of State. (2021). *The impactful role of faith actors in the COVID-19 pandemic*. United States Department of State. https://www.state.gov/the-impactful-role-of-faith-actors-in-the-covid-19-pandemic/

USAID. (2020). *Faith-based organizations responding to COVID-19*. USAID. https://www.usaid.gov/sites/default/files/documents/1875/FBOs_Mini-Compendium_508_tagged.pdf

Van Natta, M., Chen, P., Herbek, S., Jain, R., Kastelic, N., Katz, Evan, Struble, M., Vanam, V., & Vattikonda, N. (2020). The rise and regulation of thermal facial recognition technology during the COVID-19 pandemic. *Journal of Law and the Biosciences*, 1–17. https://doi.org/10.1093/jlb/lssa038

Van Ness, L. (2021, March 19). *For States' COVID Contact Tracing Apps, Privacy Tops Utility*. Pew Research. https://pew.org/3r1F7VN

Van Orden, K. A., Bower, E., Beckler, T., Rowe, J., & Gillespie, S. (2022). The use of robotic pets with older adults during the COVID-19 pandemic. *Clinical Gerontologist, 45*(1), 189–194. a9h.

Wells, J. (2020, May 27). *Coronavirus pandemic forces the funeral industry online*. CNBC. https://www.cnbc.com/2020/05/27/coronavirus-pandemic-forces-the-funeral-industry-online.html

Westrick-Payne, K., & Wendy Manning. (2022). *Marriage, divorce, and the COVID-19 pandemic in the U.S.* https://www.bgsu.edu/ncfmr/resources/data/family-profiles/westrick-payne-manning-marriage-divorce-covid-pandemic-fp-22-12.html

Wiederhold, B. K. (2020). Turning to faith and technology during the coronavirus disease 2019 crisis. *Cyberpsychology, Behavior, and Social Networking*, *23*(8), 503–504. https://doi.org/10.1089/cyber.2020.29191.bkw

Wienrich, C., Fries, L., & Latoschik, M. E. (2022). Remote at Court. In G. Salvendy & J. Wei (Eds.), *Design, Operation and Evaluation of Mobile Communications* (pp. 82–106). Springer International Publishing. https://doi.org/10.1007/978-3-031-05014-5_8

Wisner, B., Blaikie, P., Cannon, T., & Davis, I. (2014). *At risk: Natural hazards, people's vulnerability and disasters*. Routledge.

Xie, B., Charness, N., Fingerman, K., Kaye, J., Kim, M. T., & Khurshid, A. (2020). When going digital becomes a necessity: Ensuring older adults' needs for information, services, and social inclusion during COVID-19. *Journal of Aging & Social Policy*, *32*(4–5), 460–470. https://doi.org/10.1080/08959420.2020.1771237

Yang, C.-C., Tsai, J.-Y., & Pan, S. (2020). Discrimination and well-being among Asians/Asian Americans during COVID-19: The role of social media. *Cyberpsychology, Behavior and Social Networking*, *23*(12), 865–870. https://doi.org/10.1089/cyber.2020.0394

Young, J. (2022). *Pandemic lockdowns made rush-hour speeding, risky driving the new normal*. IIHS-HLDI Crash Testing and Highway Safety. https://www.iihs.org/news/detail/pandemic-lockdowns-made-rush-hour-speeding-risky-driving-the-new-normal

7

HEALTHCARE AND MENTAL HEALTH DURING COVID-19

COVID is a funhouse mirror that is amplifying issues that have existed forever. People are not [just] dying of COVID. They are dying of racisim, of economic inequality, and it is not going to stop with COVID.

Shreya Kangovi M.D. M.S.H.P

The pandemic presented an unprecedented challenge for the healthcare systems in the U.S. and globally. The COVID-19 virus was highly contagious and particularly severe in older adults and individuals with co-morbidities (Porcheddu et al., 2020). Accordingly, healthcare systems adapted to this highly infectious disease to minimize risk and curb the spread of the disease, specifically focused on older adults and others most vulnerable (Robbins et al., 2020; Handel et al., 2020). Elective surgeries were halted, and routine checks (and doctor visits) were moved to virtual environments using telehealth systems. The Centers for Disease Control and Prevention (CDC) website provided detailed procedures for managing healthcare providers (HCP) during COVID-19, including several documents, such as *Evaluating Healthcare Personnel with Symptoms of SARS-CoV-2 Infection; Return to Work Criteria for HCP with SARS-CoV-2 Infection; Return to Work Criteria for HCP Who Were Exposed to Individuals with Confirmed SARS-CoV-2 Infection; SARS-CoV-2 Illness Severity Criteria (adapted from the NIH COVID-19 Treatment Guidelines)* (CDC, 2022).

7.1 Factors Affecting Healthcare

Ahmed et al. (2020) examined stakeholders' perspectives and experiences of healthcare access for non-COVID-19 conditions before and during pandemic lockdowns in seven high-poverty communities

DOI: 10.1201/9781003319894-9

across countries. They reported that the fear of being diagnosed with COVID-19 prevented people from seeking healthcare. Additionally, residents had difficulty accessing certain facilities, which significantly reduced their ability to get help for non-COVID-19-related conditions.

The advancement of technologies offered opportunities for healthcare workers and patients to remotely handle non-COVID health-related issues. However, it raised concerns regarding the digital divide, as technology can widen the gap between groups because of preexisting social, economic, and political factors (Ramsetty & Adams, 2020; Fridsma, 2020; Dorsey & Topol, 2016; Kruse et al., 2018). As Fridsma (2020) mentioned, the American Medical Informatics Association (AMIA) proposed to include the digital divide as a social determinant of health in 2017. Taking into consideration of the context of social determinants of health, the digital divide occurred because of the mistrust, reimbursement tied options, inability to secure latest versions of technology, or comorbidity-linked access (Ramsetty & Adams, 2020).

7.1.1 Technology Shift for Healthcare

To respond to urgent needs digital health, technologies, and mobile applications were readily applied. Digital health tools play critical roles in changing the way care is provided (Klein, Hostetter & McCarthy, 2014). During the pandemic, digital technologies and solutions were widely adopted in healthcare organizations, including mobile apps for contact tracing, vaccination, and patient tracking. New digital solutions were developed fast (Ramsetty & Adams, 2020). For example, provider visits were offered via video conferencing, emails, mobile phone apps, voice assistants, wearable devices, chatbots, artificial intelligence (AI) powered diagnostic tools, and mobile sensors (e.g., smart watches, oxygen monitors, or thermometers) (Golinelli et al., 2020), all of which were less accessible pre-COVID. In a survey of early scientific literature, Golinelli et al. (2020) identified digital solutions for patients' needs to mitigate the influence of COVID-19 on patients and healthcare systems. In this study, patient needs included diagnosis, prevention, treatment adherence lifestyle, patient engagement and surveillance (Golinelli et al., 2020; Hermann, 2018).

Most research focused on the use of digital technologies for diagnosis, surveillance, and prevention, confirming the usefulness of such digital technologies in these measures (Golinelli et al., 2020). However, research was lacking on the use of digital technologies or solutions for lifestyle empowerment or patient engagement (Golinelli et al., 2020). In some cases, the increased use of digital technologies was difficult due to digital divide issues.

Prior to the pandemic, at least one study identified injustice issues that digital solutions contributed to because while these solutions enhanced healthcare access and quality, developers often ignored vulnerable and underserved populations. As stated by Van Winkle, Carpenter, and Moscucci (2017), "the technologies that are leaving these communities behind are the same ones that can best support them" (p. 1116). Therefore, they proposed several ways to support marginalized populations with digital technologies, such as employing analytics and management tools to offer interventions, and design features that suit different levels of digital literacy proficiency.

7.1.2 Digital Health During COVID-19

In healthcare, such terms as *telehealth*, *ehealth*, *mhealth*, *telemedicine*, and *digital health* have been widely used and often misunderstood. While all terms are related to the delivery of health services using digital technologies, they each have slightly different descriptions. Figure 7.1 shows the relationship among the different terms based on whether the tool is used primarily by the healthcare provider or the patient.

Digital health encompasses telehealth, mobile health, wearables, analytics, artificial intelligence, and genomics (Mathews et al., 2019). *Digital health* basically covers all internet-based technological applications used for health (Mahoney, 2020). The term *telehealth*, however, introduces the delivery of a variety of health services utilizing information and telecommunication technologies (Institute of Medicine, 2012; World Health Organization, 2016; Mahoney, 2020). Although *telehealth* and *telemedicine* are often used interchangeably, *telemedicine* is evolving as a subset of *telehealth*, and indicates direct provider-to-patient service. Therefore, *telehealth* is a larger umbrella term that refers to any healthcare services delivered remotely (Mahoney, 2020). The

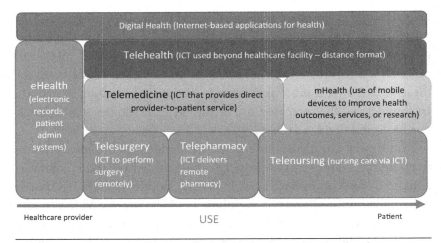

Figure 7.1   Relationship among the digital health–related terms based on the primary user.

term *mHealth* refers to the use of mobile device applications (e.g., cell phones or tablets), primarily by patients, to improve health outcomes, healthcare services, and health research (Iribarren, Cato, Falzon & Stone, 2017; Mahoney, 2020). Via mobile applications, patients and medical professionals can connect with each other to collect data needed (Iribarren, Cato, Falzon, & Stone, 2017). Finally, *eHealth* is another broader term, which specifically refers to information and communications technology used for health records, patient administration systems, and data collection; primarily used by providers in healthcare facilities (Oh, Rizo, Enkin, & Jadad, 2005).

The use of telehealth increased during the COVID-19 pandemic and was proven to reach rural populations (Ramsetty & Adams, 2020; Marcin, Shaikh, & Steinhorn, 2016). Specifically, telemedicine and remote consultation were effective to meet with non-infected patients or infected patients without symptoms (Golinelli et al., 2020). Some providers were able to remotely participate in surgeries, through telesurgery; and prescriptions were ordered online and delivered directly to patients, through telepharmacy (AlMazeedi et al., 2020; Bailo et al., 2021; Dat et al., 2022; Mohan et al., 2021; Unni et al., 2021). Telesurgery used robots, sensors, and videos to allow surgeons to participate remotely, reducing their exposure to COVID-19 (AlMazeedi et al., 2020; Mohan et al., 2021), though there were increased concerns for privacy, ethics, and legality, due to its use. Beyond the delivery of medicines, telepharmacy was used to answer patient questions, and to provide pharmaceutical education. As telepharmacy is more public facing than telesurgery, digital access and literacy were barriers to effective use (Unni et al., 2021). Globally, telenursing increased during COVID-19, where nurse-initiated phone calls to patients helped to provide continued care (Kord et al., 2021; Mamom & Daovisan, 2022). Additionally, mHealth technologies were employed during COVID-19, primarily for patients. There were over 200 mobile apps found on Google Play or the Apple App Store specifically for COVID-19 (Ming et al., 2020). Many apps were also used to mitigate the increased mental health concerns during the pandemic.

7.2 Mental Health Impacts

The twin pandemics of COVID-19 cases and the increased racism during the pandemic, exacerbated disparities and divides; and thus, in turn led to increased mental health challenges for millions of Americans. Among these Americans, marginalized populations including older adults, racial and ethnic minorities, and children had an increased risk of mental health issues (Dubois & Yuan, 2021; Dubois & Yuan, 2022). Systematic inequalities and inequities faced among the most vulnerable contributed to their mental health challenges. Vulnerability was accentuated by digital and racial divides, which caused increased mental health problems during the pandemic (Dubois & Yuan, 2021). Policies and mandates such as stay-at-home orders, social distancing, and mask wearing led to long-term mental health complications for marginalized populations (Gloster et al., 2020).

In their study examining the mental health challenges, Dubois and Yuan (2021) identified factors that influence said populations during the pandemic, and offered recommendations to assist with emergency managers, public health officials, policymakers, and academic professionals. Figure 7.2 shows the factors that affected mental health during COVID as precipitated by use (or inability to use technology). The factors included material conditions, relationship factors, personal experiences, cultural differences, and social conditions. As can be seen from Figure 7.2, the social conditions were typically the most critical factor. Under this category, communication issues such

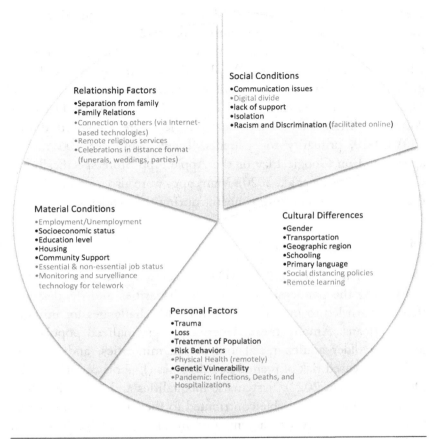

Figure 7.2   Factors and subfactors affecting the socially vulnerable populations' mental health and well-being. Created by adopting (Collis, Scott, & Ross, 2010) and the World Health Organization's depictions of the factors and subfactors influencing populations' mental health and well-being. Source: adapted from Collis et al and the World Health Organization (Collis, Scott, & Ross, 2010; Dubois & Yuan, 2021.)

as, exchanging ideas about the COVID-19 pandemic, the accentuated digital divide, the lack of support, the isolation because of the pandemic all contribute to the increased mental health challenges. Additionally, the systemic racism and discrimination caused socially vulnerable populations (particularly racial and ethnic minorities) to face inequitable healthcare and community services. Other factors in this figure include cultural differences, relationship factors, material conditions, and personal factors. As can be seen in Figure 7.2, during COVID the use of technology was prevalent in all the factors that contributed to individual mental health. However, as Dubois and Yuan (2021) pointed out, "Yet, among socially vulnerable populations who already have lower socioeconomic state, unstable unemployment, limited technology access, underlying health conditions, and face systematic injustices, addressing mental health amid a crisis becomes much harder" (p. 72).

Figure 7.2 indicates that an individual's mental health was related to such factors as relationships, employment, income, physical health, geographic location, education level, trauma, and racism, and varies across gender, race, age, and class (Dubois & Yuan, 2021; Williams, 2018).

7.2.1 Increased Racism Impact on Mental Health

It was reported that racism, xenophobia, and microaggressions were able to exacerbate mental health and led to an increased incidence of depression and suicide attempts (O'Keefe et al., 2015). During the COVID-19 pandemic, there were increased racist attacks leveraged particularly at racial and ethnic minorities, though other minority populations were at risk as well. In a study of mental health impacts during COVID by racial groups, Hispanic/Latino adults indicated the prevalence of psychosocial stress higher than other racial groups (due to food and housing insecurity) (McKnight-Eily et al., 2021). Among African Americans, the increased violence, vigilantism, and racist attacks, combined with the increased risk of infection, hospitalization, and death, contributed to mental health impacts (Chae et al., 2021; Ibrahimi et al., 2020; Novacek et al., 2020; Sneed et al., 2020). The historical impacts of systemic racism across all social determinants of health domains contributed to higher post-traumatic stress disorders among African Americans, than for other racial groups (Novacek et al., 2020). Furthermore, the prevalence of discriminatory tactics in healthcare and stigma related to mental health services led to mistrust among African Americans (Novacek et al., 2020; Sneed et al., 2020). While the first of the twin pandemics was related to infection from the COVID-19 virus, the second was due to the increased racism felt by both Asian and African American populations (Chae et al., 2021). Both populations faced increased racist attacks and had feelings of depression about the situation (Chae et al., 2021).

Asian Americans experienced anti-Asian rhetoric and stigma, which to a substantial extent have worsened their mental health issues. As Dubois and Yuan (2022) pointed out, the COVID-19 response was a political response because of the evident political divides and amplified xenophobia. It can be attributed to two reasons: (1) a lack of representation among elected leaders in government and (2) specifically blaming China for the virus caused racial discrimination and widespread xenophobia specifically toward Asian Americans and Pacific Islanders (AAPI). This sparked a social media hashtag and movement #StopAsianHate. Although AAPIs make up 6% of the U.S. population, AAPI elected leaders only occupies 0.9% across all levels of government, which is the lowest representation of any demographic (Greater Boston Staff, 2021). The lack of representation in the U.S. is a main challenge faced by Asian Americans to have a successful and equitable response.

African American populations had it particularly hard during the pandemic. The polarized police brutality during the pandemic was seemingly targeted towards African Americans, where a number of incidents were live streamed and replayed over social and broadcast media (Corpuz, 2021; Roberts, 2021; Stolberg, 2020). Ahmaud Arbery was murdered and filmed during his jog by two men aiming to make an unfounded citizen's arrest (Nguyen et al., 2021). Breonna Taylor was murdered in her home and George Floyed was murdered on the street in front of a convenience store. George Floyd's murder served as a tipping point, sparking protests. Some civilians with prior law enforcement training or aspirations thereof also targeted African Americans and the #BlackLivesMatter protests. The protests increased the exposure for so many and increased the interactions with the law enforcement monitoring the crowds. Millions of people protested in cities nationwide (Roberts, 2021). The brutality among law enforcement was seen globally, with some comparing what happened in Minneapolis to other cities worldwide (Corpuz, 2021; Jaquemet, 2021). Additionally, Black maternal health was at an all-time low, with the maternal death rate for Black women disproportionately higher compared to White or Hispanic/Latina women (Ellis & Broaddus, 2021; Hopkins Tanne, 2023). Though some deaths were related to contracting the coronavirus, the majority of deaths were not. Though all of the social determinants of health likely contributed to these outcomes, many highlighted the effect racism had on maternal health (Government Accountability Office, 2022).

Native American populations were among the hardest impacted due to the virus and the health inequities among American Indian populations (Weeks, 2021; Yellow Horse et al., 2022). Continued racism and being constantly overlooked likely contributed to the increased infection rates. In response, Tribal nations and indigenous communities developed non-profits to increase the visibility and inclusion of their voices amid Tribal nation decisions to reduce the spread (Walls, 2021). Once vaccinations became available, Navajo and Apache Nations took the lead in getting their communities vaccinated in Arizona using digital flyers (Ladyzhets/AZCIR & Montanari/AZCIR, 2023; Tang, 2022).

Several studies examined the impact of COVID-19-related racial discrimination on mental health (Chen, Zhang, & Liu, 2020; Litam, 2020; Cheah et al., 2020) and found that the mental and physical health of Black, Indigenous groups, and People of Color (BIPOC) were harmed by racism, discrimination, and microaggressions.

7.3 Digital Health for Mental Health

The twin pandemics both contributed to the increased use of mobile health apps for COVID-19 and for mental health. In a study of over 2,000 college students, the two biggest coping mechanisms for depression during the pandemic were connecting with family, friends, or loved ones and use of technologies for mental stress, 67% and 32% respectively (Wang et al., 2020). During the pandemic, mobile apps were used for COVID-19, training, and education, as well as self-assessments (Kondylakis et al., 2020).

Lui, Marcus, and Barry (2017) reviewed articles on the use of mental health mobile apps in a psychotherapy context. They focused on the effectiveness and features of such apps. Table 7.1 shows the apps included in this review. Most of the apps were stand-alone apps. Issues about anxiety/depression or substance use disorders were the major focus of these apps. Other issues, including bipolar disorders, PTSD, and schizoaffective disorder, were also addressed in mental health apps. These mental health apps gave users choices including therapeutic skills, symptom monitoring, recommendations, and psychoeducation.

Table 7.1 Mental Health Mobile Apps (Lui, Marcus, & Barry, 2017)

APP	TARGETED POPULATION	APP FEATURES	STUDY
Attention bias modification training (ABMT)	Anxiety (Undergra- duates)	Stand-alone app Serious game	Dennis & O'Toole (2014)
Cognitive bias modification of attention (CMB-A)	Social anxiety	Stand-alone app Serious game	Enock et al. (2014)
The Stress Manager	Generalized Anxiety Disorder	Adjunct • Symptom monitoring; • Menu of therapeutic skills; • Recommends therapeutic skills contingent on user response; • Positive reinforcement contingent on user response	Newman et al. (2014)
Mobilyze!	Depression	Adjunct • Symptom monitoring; • Recommends therapeutic skills contingent on user response; • Context Sensing	Burns et al. (2011)
SuperBetter	Depression	Stand-alone app • Serious Game; • Menu of therapeutic skills; • Recommends therapeutic skills contingent on user response; • Positive reinforcement contingent on user response; • Enlist social support	Roepke et al. (2015)
The Get Happy Program	Depression	Stand-alone app • Psychoeducation; • Testimonial; • Menu of therapeutic skill	Watts et al. (2013)
Improving Adherence in Bipolar Disorder (IABD)	Bipolar Spectrum Disorders	Adjunct • Psychoeducation; • Symptom monitoring; • Menu of therapeutic skills; • Recommends therapeutic skills contingent on user response; • Enlist social support	Wenze et al. (2014)
PTSD Coach	PTSD community	Stand-alone app • Psychoeducation; • Symptom monitoring; • Menu of therapeutic skills; • Recommends therapeutic skills contingent on user response; • Enlist social support	Miner et al. (2016); Possemato et al. (2016)

(Continued)

Table 7.1 (Continued)   Mental Health Mobile Apps (Lui, Marcus, & Barry, 2017)

APP	TARGETED POPULATION	APP FEATURES	STUDY
FOCUS	Schizophrenia/ Schizoaffective Disorder	Adjunct • Symptom monitoring; • Menu of therapeutic skills; • Recommends therapeutic skills contingent on user response	Ben-Zeev et al. (2014)
Location-Based Monitoring and Intervention System for Alcohol Use Disorders (LMBI-A)	Substance Use: Alcohol	Stand-alone app • Psychoeducation; • Symptom monitoring; • Menu of therapeutic skills; • Recommends therapeutic skills contingent on user response; • Context sensing	Dulin et al. (2014); Gonzalez & Dulin (2015)
Addiction-Comprehensive Health Enhancement Support System (A-CHESS)	Substance use: Alcohol	Stand-alone app • Symptom monitoring; • Menu of therapeutic skills; • Recommends therapeutic skills contingent on user response; • Enlist social support; • Context sensing	Gustafson et al. (2014)
The Brief Alcohol Screening and Intervention for College Students SmartQuit	Substance use: Smoking	Stand-alone app • Testimonial; • Symptom monitoring; • Menu of therapeutic skills; • Recommends therapeutic skills contingent on user response; • Enlist social support; • Positive reinforcement contingent on user response	Bricker et al. (2014); Heffner et al. (2015)
BASICS-Mobile	Substance use: Alcohol and smoking (undergraduate)	Stand-alone app • Psychoeducation; • Symptom monitoring; • Menu of therapeutic skills; • Recommends therapeutic skills contingent on user response	Witkiewitz et al. (2014)
mCM	Substance use: Smoking (homeless veterans)	Adjunct • Symptom monitoring; • Positive reinforcement contingent on user response;	Carpenter et al. (2015); Hertzberg et al. (2013)
DBT Coach	Substance use: (w/borderline personality disorder)	Adjunct psychoeducation • Symptom monitoring; • Menu of therapeutic skills; • Recommends therapeutic skills contingent on user response; • Enlist social support	Rizvi et al. (2011)

It seems that mental health apps were helpful in reducing primary symptoms. However, there was no substantial evidence to support that there existed one mental health app that had been experimentally validated for its effectiveness (Lui, Marcus, & Barry, 2017).

Wasil et al. (2020) analyzed 27 mental health-related apps used during COVID from the Apple App Store and Google Play Store and identified the two most popular apps, Headspace and Calm, which account for 90% of active users. Aziz et al. (2022) compared the use of mental health apps between the pre- and during COVID-19 periods in terms of age and gender of users. The users of mental health apps increased during COVID, specifically for adults over 24 years old. Men were more likely than women to use the mental health apps overall, during COVID (Aziz et al. 2022). Additionally, user engagement and retention remain the issue in use of the mental health apps.

7.4 Summary

Healthcare has experienced dramatic changes during the COVID-19. Technological advancement presented both opportunities and challenges for the general public to connect with healthcare providers. Digital solutions to healthcare include digital health, mhealth, ehealth, telenursing, telepharmacy, telesurgery and telemedicine. Due to these advancements, multiple factors contributed to the challenges, such as digital divide, social, economic, and political factors. Simultaneously, mental health issues worsened because of the twin pandemics of COVID-19 infection and increased racism. This chapter discussed mental health apps and the potential of these apps to address mental health–related issues. Further development of mobile apps for healthcare is critical to mitigate the negative impact of COVID on the sector of healthcare.

References

Ahmed, S. A. S., Ajisola, M., Azeem, K., Bakibinga, P., Chen, Y. F., Choudhury, N. N., ... & Yusuf, R. (2020). Impact of the societal response to COVID-19 on access to healthcare for non-COVID-19 health issues in slum communities of Bangladesh, Kenya, Nigeria and Pakistan: results of pre-COVID and COVID-19 lockdown stakeholder engagements. *BMJ Global Health*, 5(8), e003042.

AlMazeedi, S. M., AlHasan, A., AlSherif, O. M., Hachach-Haram, N., Al-Youha, S. A., & Al-Sabah, S. K. (2020). Employing augmented reality telesurgery for COVID-19 positive surgical patients. *Journal of British Surgery, 107*(10), e386–e387.

Aziz, M., Erbad, A., Almourad, M. B., Altuwairiqi, M., McAlaney, J., & Ali, R. (2022). Did usage of mental health apps change during COVID-19? A comparative study based on an objective recording of usage data and demographics. *Life, 12*(8), 1266.

Bailo, P., Gibelli, F., Blandino, A., Piccinini, A., Ricci, G., Sirignano, A., & Zoja, R. (2021). Telemedicine applications in the era of COVID-19: telesurgery issues. *International Journal of Environmental Research and Public Health, 19*(1), 323.

Ben-Zeev, D., Brenner, C. J., Begale, M., Duffecy, J., Mohr, D. C., & Mueser, K. T. (2014). Feasibility, acceptability, and preliminary efficacy of a smartphone intervention for schizophrenia. *Schizophrenia Bulletin,* 40, 1244–1253. http://dx.doi.org/10.1093/schbul/sbu033

Bricker, J. B., Mull, K. E., Kientz, J. A., Vilardaga, R., Mercer, L. D., Akioka, K. J., & Heffner, J. L. (2014). Randomized, controlled pilot trial of a smartphone app for smoking cessation using acceptance and commitment therapy. *Drug and Alcohol Dependence, 143*, 87–94. http://dx.doi.org/10.1016/j.drugalcdep.2014.07.006

Burns, M. N., Begale, M., Duffecy, J., Gergle, D., Karr, C. J., Giangrande, E., & Mohr, D. C. (2011). Harnessing context sensing to develop a mobile intervention for depression. *Journal of Medical Internet Research, 13*, 158–174. http://dx.doi.org/10.2196/jmir.1838

Carpenter, V. L., Hertzberg, J. S., Kirby, A. C., Calhoun, P. S., Moore, S. D., Dennis, M. F. ... Beckham, J. C. (2015). Multicomponent smoking cessation treatment including mobile contingency management in homeless veterans. *The Journal of Clinical Psychiatry, 76*, 959–964. http://dx.doi.org/10.4088/JCP.14m09053

CDC Website. Managing Healthcare Operations During COVID-19 (2022, September 23). https://www.cdc.gov/coronavirus/2019-ncov/hcp/facility-planning-operations.html

Chae, D. H., Yip, T., Martz, C. D., Chung, K., Richeson, J. A., Hajat, A., Curtis, D. S., Rogers, L. O., & LaVeist, T. A. (2021). Vicarious racism and vigilance during the COVID-19 pandemic: Mental health implications among Asian and Black Americans. *Public Health Reports, 136*(4), 508–517.

Cheah, C. S. L., Wang, C., Ren, H., Zong, X., Cho, H. S., & Xue, X. 2020. COVID-19 Racism and Mental Health in Chinese American Families. *Pediatrics, 146*(5). https://doi.org/10.1542/peds.2020-021816

Chen, J. A., Zhang, E., & Liu, C. H. (2020). Potential impact of COVID-19–related racial discrimination on the health of Asian Americans. *American Journal of Public Health, 110*(11), 1624–1627.

Collis, A., Scott, N., & Ross, D. 2010. *Workers on the move 2: European migrant workers and health in the UK: A review of the issues.* Keystone Development Trust.

Corpuz, J. C. G. (2021). 'Pandemic within a pandemic': A call to end police brutality. *Journal of Public Health (Oxford, England)*, fdab250. https://doi.org/10.1093/pubmed/fdab250

Dat, T. V., Tu, V. L., Quan, N. K., Minh, N. H., Trung, T. D., Le, T. N., Phuc-Vinh, D., Trinh, D.-T. T., Pham Dinh, L., & Nguyen-Thi, H.-Y. (2022). Telepharmacy: a systematic review of field application, benefits, limitations, and applicability during the COVID-19 pandemic. *Telemedicine and E-Health, 29*(2), 209–221.

Dennis, T. A., & O'Toole, L. (2014). Mental health on the go: Effects of a gamified attention-bias modification mobile application in traitanxious adults. *Clinical Psychological Science, 2*, 576–590. http://dx.doi.org/10.1177/2167702614522228

Dorsey, E. R., Topol, E. J. 2016. State of telehealth. *The New England Journal of Medicine, 375*(2), 154–161.

Dubois, E., & Yuan, X. J. (2021). The mental state of Americans amid the COVID-19 crisis: How socially vulnerable populations face greater disparities during and after a crisis. *Journal of Emergency Management, 19*(9), 69–80.

Dubois, E., & Yuan, X.-J. (2022). The Societal Impacts of COVID-19 on Asian Americans: Mitigating Mental Health Disparities Stemming from Labels Like the "China Virus". In "Addressing Differential Impacts of COVID-19 in NYS: A Symposium and Edited Volume" organized by Dr. Rodríguez, Dr. Bennett Gayle, Dr. Holtgrave, Dr. Pardo and Dr. Warner. SUNY Press, forthcoming.

Dulin, P. L., Gonzalez, V. M., & Campbell, K. (2014). Results of a pilot test of a self-administered smartphone-based treatment system for alcohol use disorders: Usability and early outcomes. *Substance Abuse, 35*, 168–175. http://dx.doi.org/10.1080/08897077.2013.821437

Ellis, N. T., & Broaddus, A. (2021, August 25). Black women and the pandemic: A crisis within a crisis. *CNN*. https://www.cnn.com/interactive/2021/08/us/black-women-maternal-mortality-pandemic/

Enock, P. M., Hofmann, S. G., & McNally, R. J. (2014). Attention bias modification training via smartphone to reduce social anxiety: A randomized, controlled multi-session experiment. *Cognitive Therapy and Research, 38*, 200–216. http://dx.doi.org/10.1007/s10608-014-9606-z

Fridsma, D. B. AMIA response to FCC notice on accelerating broadband health tech availability. https://www.amia.org/sites/default/files/AMIA-Response-to-FCC-Notice-on-Accelerating-Broadband-Health-Tech-Availability.pdf. Accessed April 15, 2020.

Gloster, A. T., Lamnisos, D., Lubenko, J., Presti, G., Squatrito, V., Constantinou, M., Nicolaou, C., Papacostas, S., Aydın, G., Chong, Y. Y., & Chien, W. T. (2020). Impact of COVID-19 pandemic on mental health: An international study. *PLoS One, 15*(12), e0244809. http://dx.doi.org/10.1371/journal.pone.0244809.

Golinelli, D., Boetto, E., Carullo, G., Nuzzolese, A. G., Landini, M. P., & Fantini, M. P. (2020). Adoption of digital technologies in health care during the COVID-19 pandemic: Systematic review of early scientific literature. *Journal of Medical Internet Research, 22*(11), e22280.

Gonzalez, V. M., & Dulin, P. L. (2015). Comparison of a smartphone app for alcohol use disorders with an Internet-based intervention plus bibliotherapy: A pilot study. *Journal of Consulting and Clinical Psychology, 83*, 335–345. http://dx.doi.org/10.1037/a0038620

Government Accountability Office, U. S. (2022, October 19). Maternal Health: Outcomes Worsened and Disparities Persisted During the Pandemic | U.S. *GAO*. https://www.gao.gov/products/gao-23-105871

Greater Boston Staff (Director). (2021, November 19). Asian Americans made historic strides in politics this year, but true representation still far off. In *News*. GBH. https://www.wgbh.org/news/politics/2021/11/19/asian-americans-made-historic-strides-in-politics-this-year-but-true-representation-still-far-off

Gustafson, D. H., McTavish, F. M., Chih, M. Y., Atwood, A. K., Johnson, R. A., Boyle, M. G.,... Shah, D. (2014). A smartphone application to support recovery from alcoholism: A randomized clinical trial. *Journal of the American Medical Association Psychiatry, 71*, 566–572. http://dx.doi.org/10.1001/jamapsychiatry.2013.4642

Handel, A., Miller, J. C., Ge, Y., & Fung, I. C. (2020). If containment is not possible, how do we minimize mortality for COVID-19 and other emerging infectious disease outbreaks? medRxiv preprint, https://www.medrxiv.org/content/10.1101/2020.03.13.20034892v1.full.pdf. Accessed March 25, 2020.

Heffner, J. L., Vilardaga, R., Mercer, L. D., Kientz, J. A., & Bricker, J. B. (2015). Feature-level analysis of a novel smartphone application for smoking cessation. *The American Journal of Drug and Alcohol Abuse, 41*, 68–73. http://dx.doi.org/10.3109/00952990.2014.977486

Herrmann M, Boehme P, Mondritzki T, Ehlers JP, Kavadias S, & Truebel H. (2018, March 27). Digital transformation and disruption of the health care sector: Internet-based observational study. *Journal of Medical Internet Research, 20*(3), e104 [FREE Full text] http://dx.doi.org/10.2196/jmir.9498 [Medline: 29588274]

Hertzberg, J. S., Carpenter, V. L., Kirby, A. C., Calhoun, P. S., Moore, S. D., Dennis, M. F. ... Beckham, J. C. (2013). Mobile contingency management as an adjunctive smoking cessation treatment for smokers with posttraumatic stress disorder. *Nicotine & Tobacco Research, 15*, 1934–1938. http://dx.doi.org/10.1093/ntr/ntt060

Hopkins Tanne, J. (2023). Covid-19: US maternal mortality rose during pandemic | The BMJ. *BMJ, 2023*(380), 659. https://doi.org/10.1136/bmj.p659

Ibrahimi, S., Yusuf, K. K., Dongarwar, D., Maiyegun, S. O., Ikedionwu, C., & Salihu, H. M. (2020). COVID-19 devastation of African American families: Impact on mental health and the consequence of systemic racism. *International Journal of Maternal and Child Health and AIDS, 9*(3), 390.

Institute of Medicine. (2012). *The role of telehealth in an evolving health care environment: Workshop summary.* National Academies Press.

Iribarren, S. J., Cato, K., Falzon, L., & Stone, P. W. (2017). What is the economic evidence for mHealth? A systematic review of economic evaluations of mHealth solutions. *PLoS One, 12*(2), e0170581. 10.1371/journal.pone. 0170581

Jaquemet, L. (2021, March 17). Police brutality reaches torture levels during the Covid-19 pandemic. *OMCT.* https://www.omct.org/en/resources/reports/police-brutality-reaches-torture-levels-during-the-covid-19-pandemic

Klein, S., Hostetter, M., McCarthy, D. (2014, October). A vision for using digital health technologies to empower consumers and transform the US health care system. *The Commonwealth Fund.* http://www.commonwealthfund.org/~/media/files/publications/fundreport/2014/oct/1776_klein_vision_using_digital_hlt_tech_v2.pdf?la=en. Accessed September 14, 2017.

Kondylakis, H., Katehakis, D. G., Kouroubali, A., Logothetidis, F., Triantafyllidis, A., Kalamaras, I., Votis, K., & Tzovaras, D. (2020). COVID-19 mobile apps: A systematic review of the literature. *Journal of Medical Internet Research, 22*(12), e23170. https://doi.org/10.2196/23170

Kord, Z., Fereidouni, Z., Mirzaee, M. S., Alizadeh, Z., Behnammoghadam, M., Rezaei, M., Abdi, N., Delfani, F., & Zaj, P. (2021). *Telenursing home care and COVID-19: A qualitative study.* BMJ Supportive & Palliative Care.

Kruse, C., Karem, P., Shifflett, K., Vegi, L., Ravi, K., & Brooks, M. (2018). Evaluating barriers to adopting telemedicine worldwide: a systematic review. *Journal of Telemedicine and Telecare, 24*(1), 4–12.

Ladyzhets, B., & Montanari/AZCIR, S. (2023, January 6). Community response helped reverse COVID's devastating toll on Indigenous communities in Arizona. *Arizona Mirror.* https://www.azmirror.com/2023/01/06/community-response-helped-reverse-covids-devastating-toll-on-indigenous-communities-in-arizona/

Litam, S. D. A. 2020. "'Take your Kung-Flu Back to Wuhan': Counseling Asians, Asian Americans, and Pacific Islanders with race-based trauma related to COVID-19." *The Professional Counselor,* 10(2), 144–156. https://doi.org/10.15241/sdal.10.2.144

Lui, J. H., Marcus, D. K., & Barry, C. T. (2017). It. *Professional Psychology: Research and Practice, 48*(3), 199.

Mahoney, M. F. (2020). Telehealth, telemedicine, and related technologic platforms: Current practice and response to the COVID-19 pandemic. *Journal of Wound, Ostomy and Continence Nursing, 47*(5), 439–444.

Mamom, J., & Daovisan, H. (2022). Telenursing: How do caregivers treat and prevent pressure injury in bedridden patients during the COVID-19 pandemic in Thailand? Using an embedded approach. *Journal of Telemedicine and Telecare,* 1357633X221078485. Advance online publication. https://doi.org/10.1177/1357633X221078485

Managing Healthcare Operations During COVID-19. https://www.cdc.gov/coronavirus/2019-ncov/hcp/facility-planning-operations.html. Updated February 8, 2021. Accessed October, 6.

Marcin, J. P., Shaikh, U., & Steinhorn, R. H. (2016). Addressing health disparities in rural communities using telehealth. *Pediatric Research, 79*(1–2), 169–176.

Mathews, S. C., McShea, M. J., Hanley, C. L., Ravitz, A., Labrique, A. B., & Cohen, A. B. (2019). Digital health: A path to validation. *NPJ Digital Medicine, 2,* 38. https://doi.org/10.1038/s41746-019-0111-3

McKnight-Eily, L. R., Okoro, C. A., Strine, T. W., Verlenden, J., Hollis, N. D., Njai, R., Mitchell, E. W., Board, A., Puddy, R., & Thomas, C. (2021). Racial and ethnic disparities in the prevalence of stress and worry, mental health conditions, and increased substance use among adults during the COVID-19 pandemic—United States, April and May 2020. *Morbidity and Mortality Weekly Report, 70*(5), 162.

Miner, A., Kuhn, E., Hoffman, J. E., Owen, J. E., Ruzek, J. I., & Taylor, C. B. (2016). Feasibility, acceptability, and potential efficacy of the PTSD Coach app: A pilot randomized controlled trial with community trauma survivors. *Psychological Trauma: Theory, Research, Practice and Policy, 8,* 384–392. http://dx.doi.org/10.1037/tra0000092

Ming, L. C., Untong, N., Aliudin, N. A., Osili, N., Kifli, N., Tan, C. S., Goh, K. W., Ng, P. W., Al-Worafi, Y. M., Lee, K. S., & Goh, H. P. (2020). Mobile health apps on COVID-19 launched in the early days of the pandemic: Content analysis and review. *JMIR MHealth and UHealth, 8*(9), e19796. https://doi.org/10.2196/19796

Mohan, A., Wara, U. U., Shaikh, M. T. A., Rahman, R. M., & Zaidi, Z. A. (2021). Telesurgery and robotics: An improved and efficient era. *Cureus, 13*(3).

Newman, M. G., Przeworski, A., Consoli, A. J., & Taylor, C. B. (2014). A randomized controlled trial of ecological momentary intervention plus brief group therapy for generalized anxiety disorder. *Psychotherapy, 51,* 198–206. http://dx.doi.org/10.1037/a0032519

Nguyen, T. T., Criss, S., Michaels, E. K., Cross, R. I., Michaels, J. S., Dwivedi, P., Huang, D., Hsu, E., Mukhija, K., Nguyen, L. H., Yardi, I., Allen, A. M., Nguyen, Q. C., & Gee, G. C. (2021). Progress and push-back: How the killings of Ahmaud Arbery, Breonna Taylor, and George Floyd impacted public discourse on race and racism on Twitter. *SSM - Population Health, 15,* 100922. https://doi.org/10.1016/j.ssmph.2021.100922

Novacek, D. M., Hampton-Anderson, J. N., Ebor, M. T., Loeb, T. B., & Wyatt, G. E. (2020). Mental health ramifications of the COVID-19 pandemic for black Americans: Clinical and research recommendations. *Psychological Trauma: Theory, Research, Practice and Policy, 12*(5), 449–451. https://doi.org/10.1037/tra0000796

Oh, H., Rizo, C., Enkin, M., & Jadad, A. (2005). What is eHealth (3): a systematic review of published definitions. *Journal of Medical Internet Research, 7*(1), e110.

O'Keefe, V. M., Wingate, L. R., Cole, A. B., Hollingsworth, D. W., & Tucker, R. P. (2015). Seemingly harmless racial communications are not so harmless: Racial microaggressions lead to suicidal ideation by way of depression symptoms." *Suicide & Life-Threatening Behavior, 45*(5), 567–576. https://doi.org/10.1111/sltb.12150

Porcheddu, R., Serra, C., Kelvin, D., Kelvin, N., & Rubino, S. (2020). Similarity in case fatality rates (CFR) of COVID-19/SARS-COV-2 in Italy and China. *Journal of Infection Developing Countries, 14*, 125–128.

Possemato, K., Kuhn, E., Johnson, E., Hoffman, J. E., Owen, J. E., Kanuri, N., … Brooks, E. (2016). Using PTSD Coach in primary care with and without clinician support: a pilot randomized controlled trial. *General Hospital Psychiatry, 38*, 94–98.

Ramsetty, A., &Adams, C. (2020). Impact of the digital divide in the age of COVID-19. *Journal of the American Medical Informatics Association 27*(7), 1147–1148.

Rizvi, S. L., Dimeff, L. A., Skutch, J., Carroll, D., & Linehan, M. M. (2011). A pilot study of the DBT coach: An interactive mobile phone application for individuals with borderline personality disorder and substance use disorder. *Behavior Therapy, 42*, 589–600. http://dx.doi.org/10.1016/j.beth.2011.01.003

Robbins, T, Hudson, S, Ray, P, Sankar, S, Patel, K, & Randeva, H (2020). COVID-19: a new digital dawn? *Digital Health,* 6, 2055207620920083

Roberts, J. D. (2021, June 9). Pandemics and protests: America has experienced racism like this before. *Brookings.* https://www.brookings.edu/blog/how-we-rise/2021/06/09/pandemics-and-protests-america-has-experienced-racism-like-this-before/

Roepke, A. M., Jaffee, S. R., Riffle, O. M., McGonigal, J., Broome, R., & Maxwell, B. (2015). Randomized controlled trial of SuperBetter, a smartphone-based/internet-based self-help tool to reduce depressive symptoms. *Games for Health, 4*, 235–246. http://search.proquest.com/docview/16870 49472?accountid14902

Sneed, R. S., Key, K., Bailey, S., & Johnson-Lawrence, V. (2020). Social and psychological consequences of the COVID-19 pandemic in African-American communities: Lessons from Michigan. *Psychological Trauma: Theory, Research, Practice, and Policy, 12*(5), 446.

Stolberg, S. G. (2020, June 7). 'Pandemic Within a Pandemic': Coronavirus and Police Brutality Roil Black Communities. *The New York Times.* https://www.nytimes.com/2020/06/07/us/politics/blacks-coronavirus-police-brutality.html

Tang, T. (2022, May 7). Tribes credited with elevating vaccinations in rural Arizona. *AP NEWS.* https://apnews.com/article/covid-health-pandemics-public-arizona-19b7d4293982fafccbf58c5375c49f2a

Unni, E. J., Patel, K., Beazer, I. R., & Hung, M. (2021). Telepharmacy during COVID-19: A scoping review. *Pharmacy, 9*(4), 183.

Van Winkle, B., Carpenter, N., & Moscucci, M. (2017). Why aren't our digital solutions working for everyone?. *AMA Journal of Ethics, 19*(11), 1116–1124.

Walls, V. M. O. and Walls, M. L. (2021, April 2). Indigenous communities demonstrate innovation and strength despite unequal losses during COVID-19. *Brookings*. https://www.brookings.edu/blog/how-we-rise/2021/04/02/indigenous-communities-demonstrate-innovation-and-strength-despite-unequal-losses-during-covid-19/

Wang, X., Hegde, S., Son, C., Keller, B., Smith, A., & Sasangohar, F. (2020). Investigating mental health of US college students during the COVID-19 pandemic: Cross-sectional survey study. *Journal of Medical Internet Research*, *22*(9), e22817. https://doi.org/10.2196/22817

Wasil, A. R., Gillespie, S., Patel, R., Petre, A., Venturo-Conerly, K. E., Shingleton, R. M., ... & DeRubeis, R. J. (2020). Reassessing evidence-based content in popular smartphone apps for depression and anxiety: Developing and applying user-adjusted analyses. *Journal of Consulting and Clinical Psychology*, *88*(11), 983.

Watts, S., Mackenzie, A., Thomas, C., Griskaitis, A., Mewton, L., Williams, A., & Andrews, G. (2013). CBT for depression: A pilot RCT comparing mobile phone vs. computer. *BMC Psychiatry*, *13*. http://dx.doi.org/10.1186/1471-244X-13-49

Wenze, S. J., Armey, M. F., & Miller, I. W. (2014). Feasibility and acceptability of a mobile intervention to improve treatment adherence to bipolar disorder: A pilot study. *Behavior Modification*, *38*, 497–515. http://dx.doi.org/10.1177/0145445513518421

Weeks, R. (2021, October 11). New data shows COVID-19's disproportionate impact on American Indian, Alaska Native tribes. *The Hub*. https://hub.jhu.edu/2021/10/11/map-covid-19-impact-american-indian-population/

Williams, D. R. (2018). Stress and the mental health of populations of color: Advancing our understanding of race-related stressors. *Journal of Health and Social Behavior*, *59*(4), 466–485. https://doi.org/10.1177/0022146518814251

Witkiewitz, K., Desai, S. A., Bowen, S., Leigh, B. C., Kirouac, M., & Larimer, M. E. (2014). Development and evaluation of a mobile intervention for heavy drinking and smoking among college students. *Psychology of Addictive Behaviors*, *28*, 639 –650. http://dx.doi.org/10.1037/a0034747

World Health Organization. (2016). *Global health observatory data: Telehealth*. World Health Organization. https://www.who.int/gho/goe/telehealth/en. Accessed June 1, 2022.

World Health Organization. (2020). Coronavirus disease 2019 (COVID-19) Situation Report – 65, (who.int). Accessed October, 28 2022.

Yellow Horse, A. J., Yang, T.-C., & Huyser, K. R. (2022). Structural Inequalities Established the Architecture for COVID-19 Pandemic Among Native Americans in Arizona: A Geographically Weighted Regression Perspective. *Journal of Racial and Ethnic Health Disparities*, *9*(1), 165–175. https://doi.org/10.1007/s40615-020-00940-2

PART III

Unique COVID-19 Considerations and the Future Forward

8

COVID-19 MOBILE APPLICATIONS

"Those who champion the use of smartphone tracking often ignore that the countries that successfully curbed their pandemics used smartphone apps alongside rigorous testing and aggressive phyiscal-distancing measures."

M. Ryan Calo, University of Washington (2020)

COVID-19–specific mobile applications were employed to help mitigate the impacts of the virus, primarily for contact tracing or proof of vaccination. *Contact tracing*, a term specifically defined for a certain virus, was referred to locating close contacts and was not new at the time of COVID (Maccari, & Cagno, 2021; Davis, 2020). Mobile applications were leveraged to assist with contact tracing. With the use of Bluetooth, global positioning systems (GPS), and artificial technology (AI) software, applications on mobile devices were able to track the location of infected individuals to encourage people to test themselves, wear masks, and isolate appropriately.

Later in the pandemic, vaccinations became readily available. The vaccine was one shot or a series of shots, depending on the way in which it was manufactured and the pharmaceutical company disseminating such protection. Digital technologies were used to develop COVID-19 digital vaccination certificates, which provided proof that the user was vaccinated against the virus. These technologies included the use of artificial intelligence (Vaishya, Javaid, Khan, & Haleem, 2020), smart applications, Internet of Things, Internet of Medical Things, big data, 5G/6G technology (Mbunge, 2020), geographical information systems (GIS) (Mbunge, Akinnuwesi, Fashoto, Metfula, & Mashwama, 2020), cloud computing, and Blockchain technology (Mbunge, Fashoto, & Batani, 2021).

In this chapter, the two primary uses of COVID-19 mobile applications are reviewed, providing an overview of their use, evaluation of

DOI: 10.1201/9781003319894-11

popular apps, and impacts of use among certain populations. Mobile applications were used for other healthcare needs, such as for mental health services, discussed in Chapter 7.

8.1 Contact Tracing

During the Ebola virus disease (EVD) outbreak, contact tracing was for epidemic control (WHO, 2015). Similar contact tracing was employed to mitigate the transmission of the SARS-CoV-2 (COVID-19) virus during the pandemic (Fairchild et al., 2020; Wacksman, 2021). Contact tracing emerged as a basic and necessary mitigation strategy to minimize the spread of COVID-19. Both public and private sector employers tried to track and control the disease's spread in their workplaces, which stimulated technological innovation that raised a significant amount of privacy and ethical concerns (Scassa, 2021). Researchers questioned if mobile apps for contact tracing were necessary (Soltani, Calo, & Bergstrom, 2020). In a study to assess contact tracing basics, Maccari and Cagno (2021) reported that the scientific evidence of advantages of a contact tracing app to help curb the spread of the virus was lacking; suggesting that the deployment of the privacy-invasive measure be revisited. However, they also proposed that the integration of the highest standards of privacy in a contact tracing app would be helpful to raise awareness and promote modifications in individual behavior.

8.1.1 Contact Tracing Mobile Apps

Mobile contact tracing apps provided an opportunity to carry out the task of tracing potentially infectious people in real time. For example, countries such as China, South Korea, and Singapore used these apps in which different combinations of GPS, Bluetooth, and Wi-Fi signals were used to identify people and warn those who may have been in contact with confirmed COVID-19 cases (Huang, Sun, & Sui, 2020). In the U.S., federal and state governments employed voluntary contact tracing apps (often separately) to help mitigate the spread of COVID-19. GPS and Bluetooth were the most utilized and practical technologies for contact-tracing apps (Ahmed et al., 2020). However, the adoption rates of contact tracing apps were low, which hindered such apps from reaching their maximum potential (Li et al., 2021). One of the major challenges to make such apps widely used was related to policies, in which individuals voluntarily participated and the apps were not nationally developed or encouraged. Additionally, such factors as cultural differences and social rules also contributed to an individual's decision to employ these apps.

Regardless of the varying public policy efforts, these apps were not fully effective due to public concerns over data privacy (Russo et al., 2021). Some features of COVID-19 contact tracing apps should have been reconsidered, including the accuracy of positioning and users' privacy. Major concerns included questions about the usefulness and the privacy of individual data, which could have affected mass acceptance (Akinbi, Forshaw, & Blinkhorn 2021), and perception about human rights abuses (Toh & Brown, 2020). The human rights abuses originated from the concern of potentially normalizing digital contact tracing beyond COVID-19 (Toh & Brown, 2020).

Motivation to use these apps was related to app design and individual differences (Li et al. 2021). Li et al. (2021) conducted a national survey in the U.S. to assess the impact of app design choices and individual differences on COVID-19 contact-tracing app adoption intentions. Their results indicated that individual differences including prosocialness, COVID-19 risk perceptions, privacy concerns, technology readiness, and demographics were more critical than app design choices (such as decentralized vs. centralized design), location use, app providers, or the presentation of security risks. Specifically, individuals who were more prosocial, perceived the virus as a personal risk, and had higher technology readiness were significantly more likely to install and use contact-tracing apps. Older people and essential workers were less likely to use COVID-19 contact-tracing apps, although they were among those at higher risk. Additionally, some app designs exacerbated the differential preferences among various sub-populations. For example, people living in rural areas were less likely to use the apps developed by a private industry than those developed by state health authorities. A qualitative study on the use of contact tracing apps in NY identified a connection to mental health concerns, where users were less inclined to use to app as it worsened feelings of depression, anxiety, and distress (Bennett Gayle et al. 2023). Table 8.1 shows the COVID contact tracing apps in the U.S. As can be seen from the table, each state has its own COVID contact tracing apps, which made the assessment of the effectiveness of such apps challenging.

Table 8.1   List of COVID-19 Contact Tracing Apps in the U.S. (MIT Technology Review Covid Tracing Tracker, source Li et al., 2020)

STATE	APPS	LOCATION BASED TECHNOLOGIES ENABLED
	GAEN[a]	Google App
Rhode Island	. Crush Covid RI	GPS, Bluetooth
Puerto Rico	Rastrea el Virus	Bluetooth, Google-Apple
Pennsylvania	Covid Alert PA	Bluetooth, Google-Apple
Washington	WA Notify	Bluetooth, Google-Apple
California	CA COVID Notify	Bluetooth, Google-Apple
Colorado	CO Exposure Notifications	Bluetooth, Google-Apple
Connecticut	Covid Alert CT	Bluetooth, Google-Apple
D.C.	DC CAN	Bluetooth, Google-Apple
Maryland	MD Covid Alert	Bluetooth, Google-Apple
Arizona	Covid Watch Arizona	Bluetooth, Google-Apple
South Carolina	South Carolina Safer Together	Bluetooth, Google-Apple
Oregon	Oregon Exposure Notifications	Bluetooth, Google-Apple
North Dakota	Care19 Alert	Bluetooth, Google-Apple API
Louisiana	COVID Defense	Bluetooth, Google-Apple
Michigan	MI Covid Alert	Bluetooth, Google-Apple
Virginia	COVIDWISE	Bluetooth, Google-Apple
Utah	Utah Exposure Notification	Bluetooth, Google-Apple
Wisconsin	WI Exposure Notification	Bluetooth, Google-Apple
South Dakota	Care19 Diary	Location
Wyoming	Care19 Alert	Bluetooth, Google-Apple
Hawaii	AlohaSafe Alert	Bluetooth, Google-Apple
Guam	Guam Covid Alert	Bluetooth, Google-Apple
North Dakota	Care19 Diary	Location
New Jersey	Covid Alert NJ	Bluetooth, Google-Apple
New York	Covid Alert NY	Bluetooth, Google-Apple
Alabama	GuideSafe	Bluetooth, Google-Apple
Delaware	Covid Alert DE	Bluetooth, Google-Apple
Minnesota	COVIDawareMN	Bluetooth, Google-Apple
Nevada	Covid Trace	Bluetooth, Google-Apple
New Mexico	NM Notify	Bluetooth, Google-Apple
North Carolina	SlowCovidNC	Bluetooth, Google-Apple
Wyoming	Care19 Diary	Location

[a] Google Apple Exposure Notification (see 8.1.2) was produced by a collaboration among private industry, many of the state related apps leveraged the GAEN system.

8.1.2 Private Sector – Google Apple Exposure Notification (GAEN) System

Technology companies have made several efforts to identify solutions for new challenges since the start of the pandemic. For example, they coordinated with the public health authorities to execute contact-tracing to mitigate the spread of the COVID-19. Additionally, they considered how to balance the tension between technological capacity and human rights, with particular issues related to privacy, trust, and ethics (Ness, 2021; Scassa, 2021). The collection of data of individuals from these apps, however, raised unavoidable privacy issues.

As Scassa (2021) pointed out, due to the shortcomings of manual contact-tracing systems (e.g., under-resourced public health professionals, and the need to identify contacts in more anonymous public environment), there is a demand to develop purpose-specific technologies for contact-tracing to curb the spread of the virus. Starting from June 2020, Test & Trace Corps (2022) collaborated with doctors, public health professionals, and community leaders to mitigate the transmission of COVID–19 in NYC (New York City). In 2021, New York State launched the COVID Alert NY mobile app which worked alongside the Exposure Notification developed by Google and Apple Inc.

Google and Apple announced their Google Apple Exposure Notification (GAEN) system on April 10, 2020. The GAEN system relied on Bluetooth and provided a high-level privacy protection by getting privacy experts involved, while offering a foundation for governments to create their own exposure notification apps for iOS and Android smartphones (Scassa, 2021). The GAEN system employed the smartphone's Bluetooth signal to reveal whenever two app users are near each other — normally within 2 meters for more than 15 minutes (Lewis, 2021). This app notified users of possible exposure to people infected with COVID-19 and was considered privacy-enhancing because of its decentralized data storage, and the removal of contact information after 14 days.

Based on a Pew Research Center survey of U.S. adults carried out on April 7–12, 2020, results indicated that about 60% of Americans thought that the government tracking individuals' locations through cellphones would not help limit the spread of the virus (Anderson &

Auxier, 2020). Given the voluntary participation component of these apps in the U.S., successful use was also connected to awareness. In a study on COVID Alert NY, the majority of their 65 interview participants or 249 survey respondents were not aware that the app existed or had ever used it (Bennett Gayle 2023; Yuan et al. 2022). Specifically, 45% of survey respondents had never used the app. Of the few that were aware, they worked for public health agencies or were asked to use the app by their employer or university.

8.1.3 Evaluation of Contact Tracing Apps

As Mbunge (2020) pointed out, because of the limited time for design and development, it was challenging for contact tracing apps to coordinate, integrate and synchronize a digital response at regional, state, and international levels. For example, a digital tool developed by WHO referred to as "Waze for COVID-19" was not widely accepted and therefore could not meet the expected outcomes (Strickland, 2020).

Researchers noticed the importance of evaluation of the effectiveness of CT/EN apps (Colizza et al., 2021; Yuan et al., 2022; Scassa, 2021; Lewis, 2021). Early evaluations of CT/EN apps have employed simulations to evaluate the effectiveness of the apps (Lewis, 2021). These early evaluations included the National Health Service (NHS) COVID-19 app in England and Wales, Spain's Radar Covid app, and SwissCovid app. Such evaluations showed that these apps are useful, but barriers exist. It would have been important to integrate them into local healthcare systems in appropriate ways (Lewis, 2021).

Previous research found that the data collected from the mobile phone apps posed the most risks for women, girls, and marginalized populations (Davis, 2020). There is an increased importance to consider laws and policies to protect the rights of marginalized populations when designing digital contact tracing apps (Davis, 2020). There were two possible reasons that digital contact tracing for COVID-19 could worsen inequality, including (1) unproven technologies could exacerbate vulnerabilities, and (2) tracking could open new forms of surveillance further marginalizing certain groups (Toh & Brown, 2020).

For example, many homeless adults in the U.S. who have phones may either not be able to afford the cost of digital plans or change their numbers or cell phones very often. Therefore, it is not realistic to link each user to a unique phone number, which can complicate the process of digital contact tracing (Toh & Brown, 2020). Further, Toh and Brown (2020) addressed that digital contact tracing may be harmful to the rights of disadvantaged groups because of the possibility of producing inaccurate or misleading data that compromises the public-health response, and a high rate of false negatives could cause some misleading relaxation of social distancing practices.

In a study examining the use of COVID-19-related apps for contact tracing deployed in New York State (NYS), Yuan, et al. (2022) have tried to identify differences in perception, adoption, or privacy concerns among racial and ethnic populations and across age groups. They adopted the Antecedent-Privacy Concerns-Outcomes (APCO) framework and the perceived usefulness construct and collected data from 120 Amazon Mechanical Turkers located in NYS. Specifically, with regard to the seriousness in which the pandemic was perceived by respondents, Asian and Black respondents indicated more serious perception than those of other races. Additionally, the perceived helpfulness and usefulness of the contact tracing mobile applications were closely aligned by race. With regard to privacy concerns, Asian respondents indicated less privacy concerns with use of the contact tracing mobile application, while Black respondents had more privacy concerns with the mobile app. Age was a key factor, as well. The youngest age group, 18–24, indicated the least willingness to use the app. The results of this study indicated that race and gender were critical factors to be considered regarding the use of contact tracing apps in NYS.

8.2 Proof of Vaccination Apps

Mobile apps were also developed for COVID-19 digital vaccination certificates. The certificates allowed proof of vaccination through personal mobile devices. For example, the Excelsior Pass, provided by NYS, provided proof of vaccination and negative test results, and was connected to vendor apps to securely verify the information. Similar to contact tracing apps, COVID-19 digital vaccination apps had problems with wide-scale adoption because (1) of a lack of ICT supporting infrastructure, consistent and synchronized development standards and the standardized COVID-19 vaccination certificates;

Table 8.2   List of COVID-19 Digital Vaccination Certificate Apps

APP NAME	DEVELOPER
Docket	NJ Department of Health
Excelsior Pass	NY State Department
Clear Health Pass	Hawaii
CommonPass	The Commons Project and the World Economic Forum
VeriFly	Daon (private company)
Clear: Health Pass	Clear Health Pass Holdings, LLC
IATA Travel Pass	The International Air Travel Association
VaxYes	GoGetDoc
VaccTrack	VaccTrack Inc.

Source: (Di Valentino, 2021.)

(2) socioeconomic disparities; (3) security risks and privacy; (4) of lack of framework, global standards, and policies leading to the integration and synchronization of digital solutions and data sharing; and (5) ethical concerns (Mbunge, 2020). Table 8.2 lists some of the vaccination apps available in the U.S. in 2021, with developers and vendors listed (DiValentino, 2021).

8.2.1 *Vaccination Hesitancy*

During the pandemic, the rapid development of vaccinations and the digital certificate mobile apps affected uptake of both (Forman, Shah, Jeurissen, Jit, & Mossialos, 2021), which in turn could have threaten the effectiveness of vaccines in controlling the pandemic (Newman, 2022). Vaccination hesitancy (VH) was identified by WHO as one of top 10 threats to global health (WHO, 2019). VH was defined by the WHO Strategic Advisory Group of Experts on Immunization (SAGE) as a delay in acceptance or refusal of a particular vaccine (MacDonald, 2015; Cascini et al., 2021; Nguyen et al. 2022). Newman (2022) mentioned that marginalization-generated structural and social disparities affected some populations, making them less likely to be vaccinated. There were also politically and religiously motivated anti-vaxxers who were less likely to get vaccinated (Milligan et al. 2022).

Because of the digital divide, marginalized populations may not have accessed mobile apps that generate digital certificates (Hall, Studdert, 2020). The gap between ICT access and utilization among marginalized populations made it impossible to have the COVID-19 digital vaccination certificates widely accepted (Georgieva, Beaunoyer, & Guitton, 2021). Not to mention the already well-known global socioeconomic disparities between developed and developing countries. These disparities significantly influenced the rollout of COVID-19 digital certificates because of poor internet services, infrastructure, and technical facilities (Mbunge, 2020).

8.3 Summary

Contact tracing and vaccination have been adopted as an effective strategy to curb the spread of infectious viruses. During the COVID-19 pandemic, technology companies developed and implemented contract tracing apps and digital vaccination certificates to help track the status of the exposure to COVID-19 of individuals to mitigate the spread of the virus. But these mobile apps caused concerns about privacy and security and exacerbated the preexisting disparities of socially vulnerable populations. Therefore, it is necessary to consider solutions to balance the need for mitigating the virus' spread and ensuring the privacy and ethical considerations of individuals.

References

Ahmed, N., Michelin, R. A., Xue, W., Ruj, S., Malaney, R., Kanhere, S. S., Seneviratne, A., Hu, W., Janicke, H., & Jha, S. K. (2020). A survey of COVID-19 contact tracing apps. *IEEE Access, 8*, 134577–134601.

Akinbi, A., Forshaw, M., & Blinkhorn, V. (2021). Contact tracing apps for the COVID-19 pandemic: A systematic literature review of challenges and future directions for neo-liberal societies. *Health Information Science and Systems, 9*(1), 18. https://doi.org/10.1007/s13755-021-00147-7

Anderson, M., & Auxier, B. (2020, April 16). Most Americans don't think cellphone tracking will help limit COVID-19, are divided on whether it's acceptable. https://www.pewresearch.org/fact-tank/2020/04/16/most-americans-dont-think-cellphone-tracking-will-help-limit-covid-19-are-divided-on-whether-its-acceptable/. Accessed October 4, 2022.

Cascini, F., Pantovic, A., Al-Ajlouni, Y., Failla, G., & Ricciardi, W. 2021. Attitudes, acceptance and hesitancy among the general population worldwide to retrieve the COVID-19 vaccines and their contributing factors: A systematic review. *EClinicalMedicine, 40*, 101113. pmid:34490416

Colizza, V., Grill, E., Mikolajczyk, R., Cattuto, C., Kucharski, A., Riley, S., Kendall, M., Lythgoe, K., Bonsall, D., Wymant, C., & Fraser, C. (2021). Time to evaluate COVID-19 contact-tracing apps. *Nature Medicine*, *27*(3), 361–362.

Bennett Gayle, D., Yuan, X., Dadson, Y., & Edwards, N. (2023). Contact tracing mobile application in New York: Qualitative study on the use and privacy perceptions. *Proceedings of 20th Annual Global Conference on Information Systems for Crisis Response and Management (ISCRAM 2023)* Omaha, NE May 27–31, 2023.

Davis, S. L. (2020). Contact tracing apps: Extra risks for women and marginalized groups. *Health and Human Rights Journal, 4*. https://www. hhrjournal.org/2020/04/contact-tracing-apps-extra-risks-for-women-and-marginalized-groups/

DiValentino, A. (2021, August 2). Proof of COVID-19 vaccination is required at some music venues, sports arenas, and airlines — these are the best vaccine passport apps to download. https://www.insider.com/guides/health/best-vaccine-passport-apps#vaccine-passport-apps-currently-available-1

Fairchild, A. L., Gostin, L. O., & Bayer, R. (2020). Contact tracing's long, turbulent history holds lessons for COVID-19. Contact Tracing's Long, Turbulent History Holds Lessons for COVID-19. https://news.osu.edu/contact-tracings-long-turbulent-history-holds-lessons-for-covid-19/. Accessed April 15, 2022.

Forman, R., Shah, S., Jeurissen, P., Jit, M, & Mossialos, E. (2021). COVID-19 vaccine challenges: What have we learned so far and what remains to be done? *Health Policy*, *125*(5), 553–567. pmid:33820678

Georgieva, I., Beaunoyer, E., & Guitton, M. J. (2021). Ensuring social acceptability of technological tracking in the COVID-19 context. *Computer Human Behaviour*, *116*, 106639. https://doi.org/10.1016/j.chb.2020.106639

Hall, M. A., & Studdert, D. M. 2020. Privileges and immunity certification during the COVID-19 pandemic. *JAMA*. https://doi.org/10.1001/jama.2020.7712

Huang, M., Sun, M., & Sui, Y. (2020). How digital contact tracing slowed COVID-19 in East Asia. *Harvard Business Review*. https://hbr.org/2020/04/how-digital-contact-tracing-slowed-covid-19-in-east-asia?fbclid=IwAR2co2xcEY3M68kk3qO7ht_fOsIU09XyjW8qlyY_krNFEJLyF8XFX9hYskI. Accessed November 11, 2022.

Lewis, D. (2021). Contact-tracing apps help reduce COVID infections, data suggest. *Nature*, *591*(7848), 18–19. https://www.nature.com/articles/d41586-021-00451-y. Accessed 15 March 2021; Pablo Rodríguez et al, 'A PopulationBased Controlled Experiment Assessing the Epidemiological Impact of Digital Contact Tracing' (2021) 12 Nature Communications.

Li, T., Cobb, C., Yang, J. J., Baviskar, S., Agarwal, Y., Li, B., Bauer, L., & Hong, J. I. (2021). What makes people install a COVID-19 contact-tracing app? Understanding the influence of app design and individual difference on contact-tracing app adoption intention. *Pervasive and Mobile Computing*, *75*, 101439.

Maccari, L., & Cagno, V. (2021). Do we need a contact tracing app?. *Computer Communications*, *166*, 9–18.

MacDonald NE, SAGE Working Group on Vaccine Hesitancy. (2015). Vaccine hesitancy: Definition, scope and determinants. *Vaccine*, *33*(34), 4161–4164. pmid:25896383

Mbunge, E. (2020). Integrating emerging technologies into COVID-19 contact tracing: Opportunities, challenges and pitfalls. *Diabetes & Metabolic Syndrome: Clinical Research & Reviewsht*. https://doi.org/10.1016/j.dsx.2020.08.029.

Mbunge, E., Akinnuwesi, B., Fashoto, S. G., Metfula, A. S., & Mashwama, P. (2020). A critical review of emerging technologies for tackling COVID-19 pandemic. *Human Behavior and Emerging Technologies*. https://doi.org/10.1002/hbe2.237

Mbunge, E., Fashoto, S., & Batani, J. (2021). COVID-19 digital vaccination certificates and digital technologies: lessons from digital contact tracing apps. Available at SSRN 3805803.

Milligan, M. A., Hoyt, D. L., Gold, A. K., Hiserodt, M., & Otto, M. W. (2022). COVID-19 vaccine acceptance: Influential roles of political party and religiosity. *Psychology, Health & Medicine*, *27*(9), 1907–1917.

Ness, V. Lindsay (2021, March 19). For States' COVID Contact Tracing Apps, Privacy Tops Utility. STATELINE ARTICLE. https://www.pewtrusts.org/en/research-and-analysis/blogs/stateline/2021/03/19/for-states-covid-contact-tracing-apps-privacy-tops-utility. Accessed October 5, 2022.

Newman, P. A., Reid, L., Tepjan, S., Fantus, S., Allan, K., Nyoni, T., Guta, A., & Williams, C. C. (2022). COVID-19 vaccine hesitancy among marginalized populations in the US and Canada: Protocol for a scoping review. *PLoS One*, *17*(3), e0266120.

Nguyen, L. H., Joshi, A. D., Drew, D. A., Merino, J., Ma, W., Lo, C-H., Kwon, S., Wang, K., Graham, M.S., Polidori, L., & Menni, C. 2022. Self-reported COVID-19 vaccine hesitancy and uptake among participants from different racial and ethnic groups in the United States and United Kingdom. *Nature Communications*, *13*(1), 636. pmid:35105869

Rothfeld, M., Sengupta, S., Goldstein, J., & Rosenthal, B. M. (2020, March 25). 13 deaths in a day: An 'apocalyptic' coronavirus surge at an N.Y.C. hospital. *The New York Times*. https://www.nytimes.com/2020/03/25/nyregion/nyc-coronavirus-hospitals.html

Russo, M., Ciccotti, C. C., Alexandris, F. D., Gjinaj, A., Romaniello, G., Scatorchia, A., & Terranova, G. (2021, August 2). A cross-country comparison of contact-tracing apps during COVID-19. *VoxEU.Org*. https://voxeu.org/article/cross-country-comparison-contact-tracing-apps

Sato, M. (2020, December 14). Contact tracing apps now cover nearly half of America. It's not too late to use one. *MIT Technology Review*. https://www.technologyreview.com/2020/12/14/1014426/covid-california-contact-tracing-app-america-states/. Accessed October 22, 2022.

Scassa, T. (2021). Pandemic innovation: The private sector and the development of contact-tracing and exposure notification apps. *Business and Human Rights Journal*, 6(2), 352–359.

Soltani, A., Calo, R., & Bergstrom, C. 2020. Contact-tracing apps are not a solution to the COVID-19 crisis. https://www.brookings.edu/techstream/inaccurate-and-insecure-why-contact-tracing-apps-could-be-a-disaster/. Accessed October 6, 2022.

Strickland, E. (2020, March 20). *An Official WHO Coronavirus App Will Be a "Waze for COVID-19"—IEEE Spectrum*. https://spectrum.ieee.org/who-official-coronavirus-app-waze-covid19

Test & Trace Corps. (2022). Test & Trace Corps | NYC Health + Hospitals. https://www.nychealthandhospitals.org/test-and-trace/. Accessed June 7, 2022.

Toh, A., & Brown, D. (2020). *How digital contact tracing for COVID-19 could worsen inequality*. Human Rights Watch.

Vaishya, R., Javaid, M., Khan, I.H., & Haleem, A. (2020). Artificial Intelligence (AI) applications for COVID-19 pandemic. *Diabetes & Metabolic Syndrome: Clinical Research & Reviews*. This preprint research paper has not been peer reviewed. Electronic copy available at: https://ssrn.com/abstract=3805803 Preprint not peer reviewed https://doi.org/10.1016/j.dsx.2020.04.012

Wacksman, J. (2021). Digitalization of contact tracing: Balancing data privacy with public health benefit. *Ethics and Information Technology*, 23(4), 855–861. https://doi.org/10.1007/s10676-021-09601-2

WHO. (2019). *Ten threats to global health in 2019*. WHO. https://www.who.int/news-room/spotlight/ten-threats-to-global-health-in-2019. Accessed March 3, 2022.

WHO and CDC. (2015, September). World health organization and centers for disease control, *Implementation and Management of Contact Tracing for Ebola Virus Disease*. https://apps.who.int/iris/bitstream/handle/10665/185258/WHO_EVD_Guidance_Contact_15.1_eng.pdf;jsessionid=1855C0EE27129004012F32716B1AFA56?sequence=1

Yuan, X.-J., Bennett Gayle, D., Dadson, Y. and Jung E. (2022) Perception and use of COVID contact tracing mobile applications in New York State (NYS). *Proceedings of the Association for Information Science and Technology ASIS&T 2022*. https://doi.org/10.1002/pra2.746

Yuan, X.-J., Dadson, Y., Bennett Gayle, D., & Jung, E. (2022). Perception and Use of COVID Contact Tracing Mobile Applications in New York State (NYS). *The Annual Conference of the American Society for Information Science & Technology (ASIS&T 2022)*.

9

PRIVACY AND SECURITY

"We are repeatedly told that contact tracing apps and COVID-19-related surveillance are temporary measures for use until the pandemic passes. That is likely fantasy"

Woodrow Hartzog

The pervasive use of technology during the pandemic led to issues beyond the digital divide or digital equity. The way in which the technology itself was perceived or implemented was also a concern. In fact, some individuals questioned their privacy and the security of their data when forced to use various devices, mobile apps, and other software. This was especially true when using technology to connect with government agencies (see more in Chapter 7). Previous chapters focused on the various domains in which organizations pivoted to the use of broadband wireless-based technologies for the continuity of operations and services. This chapter focuses attention on the increasing concern of cybersecurity.

According to the Cybersecurity & Infrastructure Security Agency (CISA), cybersecurity is the action of protecting networks, devices, and data from unauthorized use. This unauthorized use can cause problems for governments, organizations, or individuals (CISA, 2019). Amid COVID-19, individual-level privacy and security concerns increased along with the progression of technology. Though the pandemic forced many to use, adopt, and rely on technology, the general concerns about privacy of their personal data (and its use), as well as the security of the systems (and devices) remained. And there is evidence that these concerns were not unwarranted. Both public and private sector employers actively sought ways to control the spread of the disease in their workplaces. Their efforts stimulated technological innovation, which raised a significant amount of privacy and ethical concerns (Scassa, 2021). In education, there were privacy concerns

DOI: 10.1201/9781003319894-12

regarding data protection, security breaches, and academic miscon-duct (Abu Talib et al., 2021). Furthermore, there was evidence that potential privacy and security harm may have been greater for K-12 students than for university students due to demographics and tech-nology access (Beerwinkle, 2021).

Technology use has been a long-studied topic; therefore, reviewing the factors that lead individuals to adopt and use new technologies should have been important. In the following sections, technology acceptance models are reviewed to propose considerations for future models. Additionally, a few privacy and security concerns are featured to expose concerns of marginalized populations across the domains.

9.1 Technology Adoption and Acceptance: Review of Select Models

Theory of Planned Behavior (TPB) stated that intention and subsequent behavior to use a technology is based on attitude, subjective norm, and perceived behavioral control (Ajzen, 1991, 2011; Godin & Kok, 1996). While the attitude about the new behavior may be positive or negative, the subjective control related to the perception of social expectations of the behavior. Finally perceived behavior control reflected how difficult or easy it is to perform the behavior. TPB has been used to explore health-related behaviors (Godin & Kok, 1996) and in many ways tech-nology acceptance models reflect the initial factors explored in TPB.

The *Technology Acceptance Model* (TAM) theorized that behavioral intention and therefore use of technology is based on the attitude of the intended user (Davis, 1989). The focus was on the user's percep-tions, where attitude is explained as the intended user's perceived use-fulness or perceived ease of use of the technology. The initial theory was developed in response to the increase in technological tools to aid in job performance, such as email. Adjustments were made to the TAM model since 1989; version 2, and version 3.

Though the original TAM model explained about 40% of the vari-ance in use of certain technologies, TAM 2 model was developed to explore key determinants of perceived usefulness. The TAM 2 model extended the original model to include the subjective norm, experi-ences, voluntariness of the user, as well as the image, job relevance, output quality, and demonstrated results of the technology, which fed into the perceived usefulness and intention to use the technology

(Venkatesh & Davis, 2000). This newer model focused again on job performance in studies by Venkatesh and Davis (2000) and explained up to 60% of the variance in user intentions.

In another variation of the model, Venkatesh and Bala (2008) combined the TAM 2 model with the model of determinants of perceived use to create TAM 3. The TAM 3 model further extended the TAM 2 model to include factors that fed into the perceived ease of use, including computer self-efficacy, perception of external control, computer anxiety, computer playfulness, perceived enjoyment, objective usability (Venkatesh & Bala, 2008), in which the model started to include some privacy and security-related factors.

The *Unified Theory of Acceptance and Use of Technology* (UTAUT) posited that use was a factor of behavioral intention and facilitating conditions, where effort expectancy, performance expectancy, and social influence fed into behavioral intention (Venkatesh et al., 2003). This model also began to factor in how some demographics of the user such as gender, age, experience, influence behavior intention along with voluntariness of use.

The *Antecedent Privacy Concerns Outcomes Model* (APCO) stated that privacy concerns influenced use of technology, along with trust. The model also posited that certain antecedents such as privacy experiences and awareness, personality, and demographic differences, as well as culture or climate may influence privacy concerns (Dinev et al., 2015). A recent commentary indicated that these privacy concerns may differ based on the technology type, as well (Knight et al., 2022; Knight et al., 2023).

9.1.1 Considerations for Future Theories

From the review of the technologies used during COVID across domains in this book, other factors need to be considered. Indeed, technology type was a factor, on multiple levels. When technology was used to disseminate information, gather information on the individual, or as a bidirectional communications tool, it influenced perception and behavioral intentions. Additionally, the proprietary differences by brand and accessibility features of the technology played a role in its use, beyond the individual behavioral intention. The job relevance of the tool influenced perception and privacy concerns.

For example, the same tool will receive varying levels of support and adoption based on type of use; whether it was used for work monitoring, government data collection, or socialization. The type of use was related to trust considerations; individuals had issues trusting the tool and issues trusting of the organization that developed the tool. This was especially true for mobile applications and other software-based technologies.

The disaster event (and variations in location-based policies) under which individuals were encouraged to use such technologies also minimized the voluntary nature of their use. Under COVID-19, many of the social distancing guidelines and other response efforts led to a reliance on information and communication technologies and forcing their use unto the public. These guidelines differed by location, and therefore, one might infer that use and availability of some technologies also differed based on the location of the users. Finally, there was variation across individuals in their trust and belief about the reality of the SARS-CoV2 virus, especially in the U.S. (Bierwiaczonek et al., 2020). Individuals that regarded the pandemic as a hoax may have been less likely to adopt mobile app contact tracing technologies. Connecting these theories with the vulnerability-related theories mentioned in Chapter 1 suggests that use, availability, and accessibility of technologies during the pandemic differed among the most marginalized members of our society. Furthermore, the misinformation and trust in the reality of COVID-19 led to inappropriate protective measures and likely reduced the use of certain technologies amid the pandemic.

9.1.2 Privacy and Security Concerns Across Domains

Use and adoption of certain technologies were influenced by privacy and security concerns, for both individuals and organizations. Interestingly, there were further differences in the use of the same technology, across different domains. For example, privacy and security concerns with the use of video conferencing differed in an educational, recreational, or health setting. Some were more apt to use certain software for socializing or education, but not interested in using it in a healthcare setting. The following sections discuss some of the privacy and security challenges across some of the different social determinants of health domains.

9.1.3 Education

The use of technology for remote education during the pandemic put a strain on both students and teachers, in terms of digital literacy and curriculum rigor. However, there were additional technology concerns surrounding data privacy and security. For example, Zoombombing infringed on privacy and security, forcing a change in privacy policy standards for Zoom, a video conferencing software used by many schools for remote instruction (Elmer et al., 2021; C. S. Lee, 2021; Ling et al., 2021; Newlands et al., 2020). Through this breach in security, individual actors join in video conferencing meetings and harass participants (Ling et al., 2021). The breach typically took on three types: (1) lewd and offensive, (2) hackers, and (3) university jokes and pranks (Elmer et al., 2021). The lewd and offensive type of Zoombombing included elements of targeted hate attacks, using Zoom as a cyberhate tool (Lee, 2021). The targeted individuals were often racial and ethnic minorities, African Americans, Asian Americans, and Jewish Americans, among others (Lee, 2021; Nakamura et al., 2021). This use of technology further highlights elements of the "twin pandemics" mentioned in Chapter 7. While Zoombombing could be found across education levels, privacy breach, academic misconduct, and data protection were among the top concerns at IHEs (Abu Talib et al. 2021). Among elementary and secondary education, potential privacy and security harm varied across educational levels (Beerwinkle, 2021).

9.1.4 Employment

Employees that worked from home experienced increased digital surveillance from employers, such as screen capturing, such as Sneek, which takes periodic photos of the individual (Newlands et al., 2020). Other digital monitoring included geolocating the employee, tracking the network access, and following work email (Vitak & Zimmer, 2021). As the tools for digital workplace surveillance grew over the pandemic, so did concerns around ethics and oversight. Some researchers predicted the potential for an increase in fraud because of the use of these technologies (De' et al., 2020). Furthermore, there was an impact on human resources. For example, the remote work (and surveillance at home) also led to feeling so withdrawn, lack of control, and violations of privacy. All of these also contributed to increased mental health issues.

9.1.5 Healthcare

The rise of digital health (including telehealth and e-health) increased the potential for privacy and security concerns, as well (Jalali et al., 2021). The Department of Health and Human Services (DHHS) lifted restrictions for mobile applications to allow for their use in healthcare during the pandemic. Services such as Zoom, mentioned above – used for educational purposes – were also allowed to be used for provider-patient communication. This permitted the potential for Zoombombing to occur in the healthcare setting, but here, health information would also be compromised.

Ransomware attacks increased during the pandemic, often targeting healthcare facilities. The definition of ransomware is when data is locked and held at ransom until such time as a fee is paid to the attackers (Jalali et al., 2021). This type of attack compromised patients' health and health data.

9.1.6 COVID-19 Mobile Apps

Many of the concerns around contact tracing applications were focused on privacy, transparency, and data security (Cho et al., 2020). However, there was also a vulnerability concern among marginalized populations (Hendl et al., 2020). Privacy concerns varied based on individual users, the organization responsible for the development of the app, and the features for "tracing" within the app. Some users (older adults and certain racial and ethnic minorities) had heightened concerns about privacy and security and were more risk-averse. This was especially true in terms of using innovative technology (such as mobile apps) for something that could be done in a low-tech fashion (such as with a phone call). Other users were more concerned about their trust in the organization, such as Google-/Apple-based contact tracing app (Exposure Notification) vs. State government or State Department of Health app. Finally, the privacy and security issues could have been related to the features of the contact tracing app itself – such as the use of Bluetooth or GPS to track infected persons. In one study, contact tracing apps using Bluetooth Low Energy were discussed to be vulnerable to de-anonymizing infected persons or relay-based worm attacks, at least early in the pandemic (Baumgärtner et al., 2020).

There were similar concerns with the proof of vaccination apps (and digital vaccination certificates). Interestingly, in the U.S., there was evidence that the privacy concerns differed among the same person between the use of contact tracing app and the proof of vaccination app, even if produced by the same entity. However, with the proof of vaccination app, there were additional concerns of fraud – as in a person showing a vaccination certificate and not actually being vaccinated (Georgoulias et al., 2022).

9.1.7 Government

In some states, COVID-related data that included the names of infected persons were shared with law enforcement (Gomez-Barrero et al., 2022; Guariglia, 2020; Kruesi, 2021; Molldrem et al., 2021). The concern for how this information would be used grew among several marginalized populations, including racial and ethnic minorities and recent immigrants. Given the twin pandemics simultaneously occurring (COVID and increased racism), these populations felt unduly targeted because they had little control over how their data was shared. For example, recent immigrants feared their data would be shared with immigration enforcement (Garcini et al., 2020; Ross et al., 2021).

In some ways the reliance of certain technologies by law enforcement was hindered by public health mitigation strategies. As an example, masks prohibited effective use of some facial recognition software. Additionally, hand sanitizer had a side effect of drying hands, which reduced the amount of moisture needed for select fingerprint analyses (Gomez-Barrero et al., 2022).

9.2 Summary

This chapter discussed the importance of privacy and security concerns for user perception and adoption of technologies across the social determinant of health domains. While access and digital literacy were significant challenges during the pandemic; control over personal data and perception of security also influenced technology use. The perception and use of technology also differed based on the technology type and its use across the domains. There was evidence that proprietary features may have influenced use as well.

References

Abu Talib, M., Bettayeb, A. M., & Omer, R. I. (2021). Analytical study on the impact of technology in higher education during the age of COVID-19: Systematic literature review. *Education and Information Technologies*, *26*(6), 6719–6746. https://doi.org/10.1007/s10639-021-10507-1

Ajzen, I. (1991). The theory of planned behavior. *Organizational Behavior and Human Decision Processes*, *50*(2), 179–211.

Ajzen, I. (2011). The theory of planned behaviour: Reactions and reflections. *Psychology & Health*, *26*(9), 1113–1127. Taylor & Francis.

Baumgärtner, L., Dmitrienko, A., Freisleben, B., Gruler, A., Höchst, J., Kühlberg, J., Mezini, M., Mitev, R., Miettinen, M., & Muhamedagic, A. (2020). Mind the gap: Security & privacy risks of contact tracing apps. In *2020 IEEE 19th international conference on trust, security and privacy in computing and communications (TrustCom)*, 458–467.

Beerwinkle, A. L. (2021). The use of learning analytics and the potential risk of harm for K-12 students participating in digital learning environments. *Educational Technology Research & Development*, *69*(1), 327–330. a9h.

Bierwiaczonek, K., Kunst, J. R., & Pich, O. (2020). Belief in COVID-19 Conspiracy Theories Reduces Social Distancing over Time. *Applied Psychology: Health and Well-Being*, *12*(4), 1270–1285. https://doi.org/ 10.1111/aphw.12223

Cho, H., Ippolito, D., & Yu, Y. W. (2020). Contact tracing mobile apps for COVID-19: Privacy considerations and related trade-offs. *ArXiv:2003. 11511 [Cs]*. http://arxiv.org/abs/2003.11511

CISA. (2019, November 14). *What is cybersecurity?* Cybersecurity & Infrastructure Security Agency. https://www.cisa.gov/uscert/ncas/tips/ST04-001

Davis, F. D. (1989). Perceived usefulness, perceived ease of use, and user acceptance of information technology. *MIS Quarterly*, *13*(3), 319–340. https:// doi.org/10.2307/249008

De', R., Pandey, N., & Pal, A. (2020). Impact of digital surge during Covid-19 pandemic: A viewpoint on research and practice. *International Journal of Information Management*, *55*, 102171–102171. https://doi.org/10.1016/j. ijinfomgt.2020.102171

Dinev, T., McConnell, A. R., & Smith, H. J. (2015). Research commentary—informing privacy research through information systems, psychology, and behavioral economics: Thinking outside the "APCO" box. *Information Systems Research*, *26*(4), 639–655. https://doi.org/10.1287/isre.2015.0600

Elmer, G., Neville, S. J., Burton, A., & Ward-Kimola, S. (2021). Zoombombing during a global pandemic. *Social Media + Society*, *7*(3), 205630512110 35356. https://doi.org/10.1177/20563051211035356

Garcini, L. M., Mercado, A., Domenech Rodríguez, M. M., & Paris, M. (2020). A tale of two crises: The compounded effect of COVID-19 and anti-immigration policy in the United States. *Psychological Trauma: Theory, Research, Practice and Policy*, *12*(Suppl 1), S230–S232. https://doi.org/10.1037/tra0000775

Georgoulias, D., Pedersen, J. M., Falch, M., & Vasilomanolakis, E. (2022). COVID-19 vaccination certificates in the Darkweb. *Digital Threats: Research and Practice*, 3530877. https://doi.org/10.1145/3530877

Godin, G., & Kok, G. (1996). The theory of planned behavior: A review of its applications to health-related behaviors. *American Journal of Health Promotion*, *11*(2), 87–98.

Gomez-Barrero, M., Drozdowski, P., Rathgeb, C., Patino, J., Todisco, M., Nautsch, A., Damer, N., Priesnitz, J., Evans, N., & Busch, C. (2022). Biometrics in the era of COVID-19: Challenges and opportunities. *IEEE Transactions on Technology and Society*, 1–1. https://doi.org/10.1109/TTS.2022.3203571

Guariglia, M. (2020, April 15). *Telling police where people with COVID-19 live erodes public health*. Electronic Frontier Foundation. https://www.eff.org/deeplinks/2020/04/telling-police-where-people-covid-19-live-erodes-public-health

Hendl, T., Chung, R., & Wild, V. (2020). Pandemic surveillance and racialized subpopulations: Mitigating vulnerabilities in COVID-19 Apps. *Journal of Bioethical Inquiry*, *17*(4), 829–834. https://doi.org/10.1007/s11673-020-10034-7

Jalali, M. S., Landman, A., & Gordon, W. J. (2021). Telemedicine, privacy, and information security in the age of COVID-19. *Journal of the American Medical Informatics Association*, *28*(3), 671–672. https://doi.org/10.1093/jamia/ocaa310

Knight, T., Yuan, X., & Bennett Gayle, D. (2022). Illuminating privacy and security concerns in older adults' technology adoption. *Work, Aging and Retirement*.

Knight, T., Yuan, X., & Bennett Gayle, D. (2023). Privacy concerns: a systematic review of older adults' perceptions surrounding the use of technology. *Journal of Data Protection and Privacy*, *5*(3), 1–13.

Kruesi, K. (2021, April 20). COVID-19 data sharing with law enforcement sparks concern. *AP NEWS*. https://apnews.com/article/nv-state-wire-nd-state-wire-co-state-wire-nh-state-wire-public-health-ab4cbfb5575671c5630c2442bc3ca75e

Lee, C. S. (2021). Analyzing Zoombombing as a new communication tool of cyberhate in the COVID-19 era. *Online Information Review*, *46*(1), 147–163. https://doi.org/10.1108/OIR-05-2020-0203

Ling, C., Balcı, U., Blackburn, J., & Stringhini, G. (2021). A First Look at Zoombombing. *2021 IEEE Symposium on Security and Privacy (SP)*, 1452–1467. https://doi.org/10.1109/SP40001.2021.00061

Molldrem, S., Hussain, M. I., & McClelland, A. (2021). Alternatives to sharing COVID-19 data with law enforcement: Recommendations for stakeholders. *Health Policy*, *125*(2), 135–140. https://doi.org/10.1016/j.healthpol.2020.10.015

Nakamura, L., Stiverson, H., & Lindsey, K. (2021). *Racist zoombombing*. Routledge.

Newlands, G., Lutz, C., Tamò-Larrieux, A., Villaronga, E. F., Harasgama, R., & Scheitlin, G. (2020). Innovation under pressure: Implications for data privacy during the Covid-19 pandemic. *Big Data & Society*, *7*(2), 2053951720976680. https://doi.org/10.1177/2053951720976680

Ross, H. M., Desiderio, S., St. Mars, T., & Rangel, P. (2021). US immigration policies pose threat to health security during COVID-19 pandemic. *Health Security*, *19*(S1), S-83. https://doi.org/10.1089/hs.2021.0039

Scassa, T. (2021). Administrative law and the governance of automated decision making: A critical look at Canada's directive on automated decision making. *UBCL Review*, *54*, 251.

Venkatesh, V., & Bala, H. (2008). Technology acceptance model 3 and a research agenda on interventions. *Decision Sciences*, *39*(2), 273–315.

Venkatesh, V., & Davis, F. D. (2000). A theoretical extension of the technology acceptance model: Four longitudinal field studies. *Management Science*, *46*(2), 186–204.

Venkatesh, V., Morris, M. G., Davis, G. B., & Davis, F. D. (2003). User acceptance of information technology: Toward a unified view. *MIS Quarterly*, 425–478.

Vitak, J., & Zimmer, M. (2021). Workers' Attitudes toward Increased Surveillance during and after the Covid-19 Pandemic. *Items: Insights from the Social Sciences*.

10
CONCLUSION

"It had taken eight months and I was still no closer to seeing my first telemedicine patient. Yet once COVID hit, within two weeks, we had been able to turn this whole thing around, and I am doing virtual consulting and testing. It has been amazing to see how quickly healthcare overall has been able to adjust and change and do what is right for our patients in the middle of a crisis."

Candace Westgate, D.O., founder of the Adventist Health Early All-Around Detection (AHEAD) program

There is no misunderstanding the influence technology had over all the domains identified in the social determinants of health during the pandemic. While availability of technology and digital literacy were among the first concerns, the accessibility of the hardware and software should also be considered. Furthermore, the perception of privacy and security for the technology should have also been prioritized. As Figure 10.1 shows, several factors across the domains contributed to the disparate use of technology among the U.S. population. Viewing the pandemic from a disaster science lens, the disparate use is not surprising. Preexisting inequities are often exacerbated due to the impacts of a disaster (Cannon et al., 2003; Kelman & Mather, 2008; Peacock et al., 2014; Sanderson, 2000; Thomas et al., 2009; Wisner et al., 2004). Beyond the primary impacts of the pandemic (such as infections, hospital admissions, or death), there were secondary impacts (Clay & Rogus, 2021). These secondary impacts did not cause people to get the virus. Instead, they affected economic stability, physical environment, education, safety, social connections, and access to healthcare which leads to adverse health outcomes (Dubois et al., 2022). As shown in Figure 10.1, technology influenced the ability to fully participate across the social determinants of health (SDH) domains during the pandemic. Also emphasized in Figure 10.1 is the

DOI: 10.1201/9781003319894-13

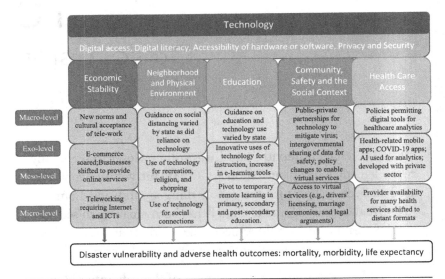

Figure 10.1   Examples of technology use amid the pandemic across the social determinants of health.

influence technology use across domains had at the individual (micro-level), community level (meso-level), business and organization level (exo-level), and with policy, norms, and culture (macro-level). Many of the technologies introduced cross over multiple levels and/or domains. This chapter serves as an overview of these secondary impacts, which may have led to a more difficult recovery, providing a conclusion for the entire book.

In the U.S., pandemic guidance varied by governments from federal to local and across local jurisdictions within the same state (KFF, 2021). This led to differences in messaging, mitigation efforts, and mandates, as most employment was categorized as essential or non-essential at the height of the pandemic. The variation in guidance contributed to differential exposure: some workers became more exposed to the virus, while others faced extreme isolation. However, technology was leveraged to minimize exposure and continue operations for essential and non-essential workers. Prior to the pandemic, technology access was often handled as a luxury. Digital inequities were very real (Budnitz & Tranos, 2022; Chang et al., 2021; Clare, 2021; Cox, 2008; Cullen, 2001; Eruchalu et al., 2021; Moldavan et al., 2022; van Dijk, 2006). High-speed internet was costly, leaving many low-income populations without access. As many disaster-related research models theorized, lack of access to communication and proper resources often hinders the recovery of marginalized populations. The access and use of technology, primarily broadband wireless information, and communications technology, during the pandemic, exposed many inequities. Post-pandemic, we should acknowledge that technology can no longer be viewed as a luxury (Budnitz & Tranos, 2022; Chang et al., 2021; Clare, 2021; Eruchalu et al., 2021; Moldavan et al., 2022). Accessible and effective technology may be key to our resilience and critical to our recovery. There were several examples of the use of technology opening doors or empowering populations. But there was also evidence that there is still a lot of work to be done to remove barriers for underserved or marginalized populations.

10.1 Opportunities for Empowerment

The policies and mandates enacted to keep people safe during COVID-19 also contributed to the increased patronage of online businesses, which benefited the e-commerce industries (Brewster, 2022; Weise, 2021). Brick-and-mortar businesses that quickly developed an online presence with the use of broadband wireless technologies (and partnerships with e-commerce corporations) ensured they were among the firms least impacted by the slowing market (Bloom et al., 2021). Empowering opportunities existed among novel businesses. New forms of entertainment were introduced, such as online music concerts and social media parties. Novel advances that were specific to the pandemic helped aid in the establishment of new businesses, as well.

Beyond businesses, the increased use of technology also benefited some households and individuals. The new near-universal telecommuting structure allowed many to experience the ever-elusive work-life balance. Among the new classifications of employment, non-essential businesses leveraged technologies for continuity of operations, especially using e-commerce apps and monitoring systems as employees worked from home. Even though there were significant supply chain issues during the pandemic, several business plan to incorporate new strategies and leveraged data analytics, artificial intelligence, and blockchain technologies, among others, in the future. In terms of the pursuit of education, many students thrived with remote instruction allowing flexibility in working at their own pace. For educational facilities at all levels, the pandemic forced innovations across modalities to facilitate learning with quality software and systems to support remote instruction.

Forehead thermometer checks, thermal cameras, and other means for remote thermal detection were used by government agencies at ports of entry to minimize the spread and increase public safety. Mobile apps were developed for contact tracing and proof of vaccination to bring awareness and encourage public health risk perception. Several innovative strategies were introduced to aid in the response, recovery, and mitigation efforts of other simultaneous disasters, such as spray grounds, automatic person counters for crowd management, software for emergency management resources, and the virtual EOC (Holdeman, 2022; Indiana University News, 2020; Rinde, 2020). Many legal services changed; marriages in some states were allowed to commence totally online; judicial hearings and trials were live-streamed; and driver's license written tests were conducted online – with some states waiving the road test during the pandemic (Baldwin et al., 2020; Crowley, 2020; Dubois et al., 2022; Feiss et al., 2021; Wienrich et al., 2022). Mobile apps and video conferencing were used to quell social isolation and attempt new hobbies (Cosco et al., 2021; Drouin et al., 2020; Eghtesadi, 2020; Kasar & Karaman, 2021; Marston et al., 2020; Van Orden et al., 2022). Curbside checkout increased in popularity as many purchases were made online. Religious ceremonies, holidays, and funerals occurred via the use of live streaming or video conferencing technologies; if they occurred at all (Burrell & Selman, 2022; Campbell, 2020; Parish, 2020; Pitsillides & Wallace, 2021; Wells, 2020; Wiederhold, 2020). The use of technology for healthcare proved transformative for some purposes. The successful use of telepharmacy may reinvent future pharmacy services (Dat et al., 2022). Telehealth technologies were able to extend the reach of healthcare providers to underserved populations.

10.2 Barriers to Use

Though there were several empowering opportunities, many populations and businesses were left behind. The twin pandemics of COVID and increased racism (and violence) further disenfranchised marginalized populations. For example, racial and ethnic minorities were among the populations most at risk due to the primary impacts of the virus. They also suffered due to the secondary impacts as well. Racial and ethnic minorities were among the groups with the highest rates of depression and stress. On top of that, racist and violent attacks targeted racial and ethnic minorities facilitated through technology during the pandemic (Bailey et al., 2022; Ruiz et al., 2020; Yang et al., 2020). Minority-owned businesses were disproportionately impacted, also.

In another example, the increased use of ICTs for business may have contributed to significant unemployment. Women left the labor force in record numbers. Simultaneously interpersonal violence increased, also disproportionately impacting women (Cappa & Jijon, 2021; Grover et al., 2021; Lund, 2020; Mazza et al., 2020; Roesch et al., 2020; Su et al., 2021).

The increased use of ICTs also opened the door to cybersecurity concerns. Ransomware attacks increased, particularly in hospital settings (Jalali et al., 2021). Despite public health efforts, COVID-19 mobile apps were not fully embraced due to data privacy concerns (Russo, 2021). Human rights issues rose due to the sharing of COVID-19-related data among law enforcement personnel and the potential normalization for the use of digital contact tracing beyond COVID-19 (Toh & Brown, 2020). Many privacy and security challenges with a virtual judicial process may have affected the protection of rights and full participation (Hershkoff & Miller, 2020; Wienrich et al., 2022).

10.2.1 Barriers across the SDH Domains

These potential barriers existed across the social determinants of health domains. Minority-, immigrant-, and women-owned businesses disproportionally suffered during the pandemic (Bloom et al., 2021; Fairlie, 2020). Business utilization of monitoring and surveillance systems for telecommuting professionals led to increased anxiety among workers. A significant number of primarily non-essential workers lost their jobs, in part due to automation (Shutters, 2021).

The stress of learning online led to anxiety and related discomforts for students. Similarly, teachers struggled to learn new technologies for pedagogical purposes, and parents were challenged trying to juggle both childcare and work. Some coursework was not easily instructed using online learning tools. Marginalized students were disadvantaged due to digital access and literacy issues. And for those reliant on other needs such as food, healthcare, and social support previously obtained at school, they had to grapple with finding replacement solutions.

Places of worship strived to keep their parishioners and maintain funding, which challenged smaller churches (Boorstein, 2020). Service providers faced several barriers, including the lack of technological access among clients and proper training (Holliday et al., 2020). Service providers also struggled to foster trust and build relationships in virtual environments with clients most in need. Similarly, trust issues influenced the public decision to use mobile apps and some telehealth technologies (Hall & Studdert, 2020). Inaccessibility to use health-related technology during this time may have contributed to unnecessary adverse health outcomes (Ramsetty & Adams, 2020).

10.2.2 Barriers Related to the Twin Pandemics

Several researchers focused on the twin pandemics: infection from COVID and increased racism during the pandemic (Bailey et al., 2022; Chae et al., 2021; Hershkoff & Miller, 2020; Ibrahimi et al., 2020; Nittle, 2020; Ruiz et al., 2020). From food insecurity, healthcare treatment, unemployment, educational inequities, and increased interpersonal violence, racial and ethnic minorities were subject to mistreatment at disproportionate rates (Bailey et al., 2022; Chae et al., 2021; Hershkoff & Miller, 2020; Nittle, 2020). Furthermore, many racist and violent attacks were facilitated through technology, primarily toward Black and Asian American populations (Bailey et al., 2022; Ruiz et al., 2020).

There is evidence racism was not the only discriminatory tactic that increased during COVID. In general, interpersonal violence increased, such as domestic violence, primarily against women and children (Cappa & Jijon, 2021; Roesch et al., 2020; Su et al., 2021). There was also an increase in discrimination and hate (particularly online) against members of the LGBTQ community (Farkas & Romaniuk, 2020). Combined with the overall impacts of the pandemic on the broader population, the twin pandemics contributed to extensive adverse health outcomes, namely, mental health struggles (Dubois & Yuan, 2021).

10.2.3 Mental Health

Although this book focused on the impacts due to the use of technology during COVID, the mental health struggles cannot be ignored. In fact, as our summary suggests, the use of technology and mental health were connected during the pandemic (Bailey et al., 2022; Ruiz et al., 2020). It is true that dealing with the primary effects of the pandemic contributed to mental health issues, as people grappled with infection rates, long hospitalizations, and deaths. However, the secondary effects also contributed to mental health issues, namely, economic instability, unsafe housing conditions, work frustrations, and learning difficulties during the pandemic. Furthermore, the increased use of technology to substitute in-person activities also contributed to mental health concerns, on top of everything else (Shutters, 2021). People struggled to gain access to the proper hardware, software, or internet to keep up with the continued pace of everyday life, including work, education, employment, government services, social services, and recreation. People also struggled to build proper connections with others, often when most critical. Furthermore, the increased discrimination, interpersonal violence, and racism that also increased during the pandemic contributed to mental well-being (Dubois & Yuan, 2021).

10.3 Going Forward: Practice, Policy, and Research

Given that some have experienced opportunities and freedoms not previously afforded to them pre-pandemic, a question about the sustainability of some of the new technologies and new uses of older technology are warranted post-pandemic. Many have been empowered by what the technology – and policies that allowed for their use – afforded them. However, as the pandemic-related mitigation strategies subside, so did the ubiquitous use of ICTs. After two plus years of working from home, many were required to return to their in-person jobs.

There has been pushback, specifically among previously telecommuting employees. This pushback is starting to create a new normal, one in which working from home is widely accepted. The pandemic created a perfect experiment to test job performance, employee satisfaction, and productivity. For some, all three of these indicators correlated positively with working from home. (Ladka, 2020; Vasel, 2021; Howe et al. 2021). Since the "experiment," many employers have either eagerly or reluctantly accommodated teleworking opportunities for much of their workforce, as many workers refuse to return to a full-time in-person job (Howe et al. 2021).

However, due to the extensive barriers to using technologies remotely, considerations must be made for those who thrive with an in-person environment. Students were excited to return to face-to-face instruction, as were instructors. Brick-and-mortar businesses that survived were anxious to get back to normal – with in-person sales. Even some of the e-commerce businesses saw their stock plummet as people returned to shopping in physical stores. Going forward, there needs to be considerations for practice, policy, and research on what it means to rely on technology, especially during a disaster.

10.3.1 Considerations for Practice

Several lessons were learned by businesses and non-profits, as they started to change procedures to include risk reduction strategies, consider ethical use of technology, and transparency. Supply chain executives are beginning to move toward risk resilience by incorporating digital technologies (Alicke et al., 2021). Similarly, hospitality industries and others will need to develop clear guidelines for telework that considers employee privacy (Chae et al., 2021). Small and medium-sized businesses, including sole proprietorship industries, should consider communications and continuity of operations plans for disasters of all hazards, which leverage a variety of technologies.

Given that the private sector's use of technology for the continuity of business operations often affects employees and clients, more careful consideration of the impacts of the digital divide is necessary. Training should be provided to employees. Technical assistance for customers should include the use of low-level technology, such as phone calls or emails, to fill in the gap when face-to-face communication is restricted.

Lessons from the social services sector encouraged all agencies to consider alternate means to build trust around marginalized communities. As these communities are often most at risk of disasters, they also face the most difficulty. Community engagement should be intentional and deliberate to determine unmet needs.

Finally, in lessons learned from several years of disaster research, emergency management and public health messaging need to be consistent across multiple modalities and technologies, as well as across agencies. Additionally, as learned from COVID-19, crafting appropriate messages should consider the potential protracted length of recovery and subsequent message fatigue.

10.3.2 Considerations for Policy

As the U.S. navigates the new normal, there are several considerations that need to be made to ensure the equitable use, access, and implementation of digital technologies. As the use of technology becomes increasingly correlated with health outcomes and disaster resilience, it will become important to keep an eye on expanding vulnerabilities. Some suggestions include the following:

- Understand where technology has empowered individuals and communities across the social determinants of health domains, as well as during disasters of all hazards.
- Investigate how technology has perpetuated digital inequities that may lead to adverse health impacts and disproportionate marginalization.
- Consider the increasing presence of technology as a staple and not a luxury.
- Incorporate training across the social determinants of health domains for businesses, organizations, government agencies, and individuals. This training should include the following:
  - Recognizing digital access
  - Increasing digital literacy
  - Inventorying accessibility features of devices and other ICTs
  - Understanding data privacy and security

10.3.3 Considerations for Research

More research should focus on technology as both a super social determinant of health and micro-level tools for all-hazards disaster resilience. Though much has been studied around the digital divide (primarily in healthcare and education), more can be investigated regarding digital access, digital literacy, accessibility features of technology, and privacy security concerns. As structured now (Figure 10.1), all the SDH domains lead to adverse health outcomes. However, less is known about the influence technology may have on economic stability, neighborhood and the physical environment, and the social context. During COVID-19, multiple modes of technology were used across all domains. In some cases, the same technology varied in use across all domains. Additionally, individual (or micro-level) impacts, facilitated by or due to the inaccessibility of technology, were identified across all domains during the pandemic. Therefore, interdisciplinary research should also address adverse health outcomes and recovery difficulties during disasters which are influenced by all SDH domains.

References

Alicke, K., Barriball, E., & Trautwein, V. (2021, November 23). *How COVID-19 is reshaping supply chains | McKinsey.* Mckinsey and Co. https://www.mckinsey.com/capabilities/operations/our-insights/how-covid-19-is-reshaping-supply-chains

Bailey, A. L., Martínez, J. F., Oranje, A., & Faulkner-Bond, M. (2022). Introduction to twin pandemics: How a global health crisis and persistent racial injustices are impacting educational assessment. *Educational Assessment, 27*(2), 93–97. https://doi.org/10.1080/10627197.2022.2097782

Baldwin, J. M., Eassey, J. M., & Brooke, E. J. (2020). Court operations during the COVID-19 pandemic. *American Journal of Criminal Justice, 45*(4), 743–758. https://doi.org/10.1007/s12103-020-09553-1

Bloom, N., Fletcher, R., & Yeh, E. (2021). *Impact of COVID-19 on US Firms [Working paper 28314].* National Bureau of Economic Research. https://www.nber.org/system/files/working_papers/w28314/w28314.pdf

Boorstein, M. (2020, April 24). Church donations have plunged because of the coronavirus. Some churches won't survive. *Washington Post.* https://www.washingtonpost.com/religion/2020/04/24/church-budgets-coronavirus-debt/

Brewster, M. (2022, April 27). *E-commerce sales surged during the pandemic.* US Census. https://www.census.gov/library/stories/2022/04/ecommerce-sales-surged-during-pandemic.html

Budnitz, H., & Tranos, E. (2022). Working from home and digital divides: Resilience during the pandemic. *Annals of the American Association of Geographers, 112*(4), 893–913. a9h.

Burrell, A., & Selman, L. E. (2022). How do funeral practices impact bereaved relatives' mental health, grief and bereavement? A mixed methods review with implications for COVID-19. *OMEGA - Journal of Death and Dying, 85*(2), 345–383. https://doi.org/10.1177/0030222820941296

Campbell, H. (2020). *Religion in Quarantine: The Future of Religion in a Post-Pandemic World.* https://oaktrust.library.tamu.edu/bitstream/handle/1969. 1/188004/Religion%20in%20Quarantine-PDF-eBook-final-2020. pdf?sequence=4

Cannon, T., Twigg, J., & Rowell, J. (2003). Social vulnerability, sustainable livelihoods and disasters. *Report to DFID Conflict and Humanitarian Assistance Department (CHAD) and Sustainable Livelihoods Support Office, 93.*

Cappa, C., & Jijon, I. (2021). COVID-19 and violence against children: A review of early studies. *Child Abuse & Neglect, 116*, 105053. https://doi. org/10.1016/j.chiabu.2021.105053

Chae, D. H., Yip, T., Martz, C. D., Chung, K., Richeson, J. A., Hajat, A., Curtis, D. S., Rogers, L. O., & LaVeist, T. A. (2021). Vicarious racism and vigilance during the COVID-19 pandemic: Mental health implications among Asian and Black Americans. *Public Health Reports, 136*(4), 508–517.

Chang, J. E., Lai, A. Y., Gupta, A., Nguyen, A. M., Berry, C. A., & Shelley, D. R. (2021). Rapid transition to telehealth and the digital divide: Implications for primary care access and equity in a post-COVID era. *Milbank Quarterly, 99*(2), 340–368. a9h.

Clare, C. A. (2021). Telehealth and the digital divide as a social determinant of health during the COVID-19 pandemic. *Network Modeling Analysis in Health Informatics and Bioinformatics, 10*(1), 26. https://doi.org/10.1007/ s13721-021-00300-y

Clay, L. A., & Rogus, S. (2021). Primary and secondary health impacts of COVID-19 among minority individuals in New York state. *International Journal of Environmental Research and Public Health, 18*(2), Article 2. https://doi.org/10.3390/ijerph18020683

Cosco, T. D., Fortuna, K., Wister, A., Riadi, I., Wagner, K., & Sixsmith, A. (2021). COVID-19, social isolation, and mental health among older adults: A digital catch-22. *Journal of Medical Internet Research, 23*(5), e21864. https://doi.org/10.2196/21864

Cox, M. (2008). Researching IT in education. In J. Voogt, & G. Knezek (Eds.), *International Handbook of Information Technology in Primary and Secondary Education*, Vol. 20. Boston, MA: Springer. https://doi. org/10.1007/978-0-387-73315-9_61

Crowley, J. (2020, April 30). Getting married online is now legal in New York. *Newsweek.* https://www.newsweek.com/project-cupid-new-york-coronavirus-weddings-online-marriage-license-1501252

Cullen, R. (2001). Addressing the digital divide. *Online Information Review*, *25*(5), 311–320. https://doi.org/10.1108/14684520110410517

Dat, T. V., Tu, V. L., Quan, N. K., Minh, N. H., Trung, T. D., Le, T. N., Phuc-Vinh, D., Trinh, D.-T. T., Pham Dinh, L., & Nguyen-Thi, H.-Y. (2022). Telepharmacy: A systematic review of field application, benefits, limitations, and applicability during the COVID-19 pandemic. *Telemedicine and E-Health*, *29*(2), 209–221.

Drouin, M., McDaniel, B. T., Pater, J., & Toscos, T. (2020). How parents and their children used social media and technology at the beginning of the COVID-19 pandemic and associations with anxiety. *Cyberpsychology, Behavior, and Social Networking*, *23*(11), 727–736.

Dubois, E., Yuan, X., Bennett, D., Khurana, P., Knight, T., Laforce, S., Turetsky, D., & Wild, D. (2022). Socially vulnerable populations adoption of technology to address lifestyle changes amid COVID-19 in the US. *Data and Information Management*, 100001. https://doi.org/10.1016/j.dim.2022.100001

Dubois, E., & Yuan, X. J. (2021). The mental state of Americans amid the COVID-19 crisis: How socially vulnerable populations face greater disparities during and after a crisis. *Journal of Emergency Management*, *19*(9), 69–80.

Eghtesadi, M. (2020). Breaking social isolation amidst COVID-19: A viewpoint on improving access to technology in long-term care facilities. *Journal of the American Geriatrics Society*, *68*(5), 949.

Eruchalu, C. N., Pichardo, M. S., Bharadwaj, M., Rodriguez, C. B., Rodriguez, J. A., Bergmark, R. W., Bates, D. W., & Ortega, G. (2021). The expanding digital divide: Digital health access inequities during the COVID-19 pandemic in New York city. *Journal of Urban Health*, *98*(2), 183–186. https://doi.org/10.1007/s11524-020-00508-9

Fairlie, R. (2020). The impact of COVID-19 on small business owners: Evidence from the first three months after widespread social-distancing restrictions. *Journal of Economics & Management Strategy*, *29*(4), 727–740. https://doi.org/10.1111/jems.12400

Farkas, K. J., & Romaniuk, J. R. (2020). Social work, ethics and vulnerable groups in the time of coronavirus and Covid-19. *Society Register*, *4*(2), 67–82.

Feiss, R., Hautmann, A., Asa, N., Hamann, C., Peek-Asa, C., & Yang, J. (2021). Balancing safety on the road with risk from COVID-19: A content analysis of policy adaptations by divisions of motor vehicles. *Accident Analysis & Prevention*, *162*, 106400. https://doi.org/10.1016/j.aap.2021.106400

Grover, S., Gupta, B. M., Mamdapur, G. M., & Surulinathi, M. (2021). Bibliometric study of publications on impact of Covid-19 and sleep disorders. *Journal of Young Pharmacists*, *13*, S72–S77. a9h.

Hall, M. A., & Studdert, D. M. (2020). Privileges and immunity certification during the COVID-19 pandemic. *JAMA*, *323*(22), 2243–2244. https://doi.org/10.1001/jama.2020.7712

Hershkoff, H., & Miller, A. R. (2020). Courts and civil justice in the time of COVID: Emerging trends and questions to ask. *New York University Journal of Legislation and Public Policy, 23*(2), 321–424.

Holdeman, E. (2022, February 1). The virtual EOC. *GovTech.* https://www.govtech.com/disaster-zone/the-virtual-eoc

Holliday, S. B., Hunter, S. B., Dopp, A. R., Chamberlin, M., & Iguchi, M. Y. (2020). *Exploring the impact of COVID-19 on social services for vulnerable populations in Los Angeles: Lessons learned from community providers.* RAND Corporation. https://www.rand.org/pubs/research_reports/RRA431-1.html

Howe, D. C., Chauhan, R. S., Soderberg, A. T., & Buckley, M. R. (2021). Paradigm shifts caused by the COVID-19 pandemic. *Organizational Dynamics, 50*(4), 100804.

Ibrahimi, S., Yusuf, K. K., Dongarwar, D., Maiyegun, S. O., Ikedionwu, C., & Salihu, H. M. (2020). COVID-19 devastation of African American families: Impact on mental health and the consequence of systemic racism. *International Journal of Maternal and Child Health and AIDS, 9*(3), 390.

Indiana University News. (2020, June 22). Free, public dashboard helps emergency managers share critical COVID-19 information. *Indiana University Information Technology News & Events.* https://itnews.iu.edu/articles/2020/Free-public-dashboard-helps-emergency-managers-share-critical-COVID-19-information-.php#:~:text=Free%2C%20public%20dashboard%20helps%20emergency,police%2C%20and%20health%20and%20medical

Jalali, M. S., Landman, A., & Gordon, W. J. (2021). Telemedicine, privacy, and information security in the age of COVID-19. *Journal of the American Medical Informatics Association, 28*(3), 671–672. https://doi.org/10.1093/jamia/ocaa310

Kasar, K. S., & Karaman, E. (2021). Life in lockdown: Social isolation, loneliness and quality of life in the elderly during the COVİD-19 pandemic: A scoping review. *Geriatric Nursing, 42*(5), 1222–1229.

Kelman, I., & Mather, T. A. (2008). Living with volcanoes: The sustainable livelihoods approach for volcano-related opportunities. *Journal of Volcanology and Geothermal Research, 172*(3–4), 189–198.

KFF. (2021, June 3). State actions to mitigate the spread of COVID-19. *KFF.* https://www.kff.org/other/state-indicator/state-actions-to-mitigate-the-spread-of-covid-19/

Ladka, Susan, (2020, April 2). These Companies Put Employees First During Pandemic. *Society for Human Resource Management.* https://www.shrm.org/resourcesandtools/hr-topics/employee-relations/pages/these-companies-put-employees-first-during-pandemic.aspx

Lund, E. M. (2020). Interpersonal violence against people with disabilities: Additional concerns and considerations in the COVID-19 pandemic. *Rehabilitation Psychology, 65*(3), 199–205. https://doi.org/10.1037/rep0000347

Marston, H. R., Musselwhite, C., & Hadley, R. A. (2020). *COVID-19 vs social isolation: The impact technology can have on communities, social connections and citizens. The British Society of Gerontology.*

Mazza, M., Marano, G., Lai, C., Janiri, L., & Sani, G. (2020). Danger in danger: Interpersonal violence during COVID-19 quarantine. *Psychiatry Research, 289*, 113046. https://doi.org/10.1016/j.psychres.2020.113046

Moldavan, A. M., Capraro, R. M., & Capraro, M. M. (2022). Navigating (and Disrupting) the digital divide: Urban teachers' perspectives on secondary mathematics instruction during COVID-19. *Urban Review, 54*(2), 277–302. a9h.

Nittle, N. (2020, May 5). *People of color are at greater risk of COVID-19. Systemic racism in the food system plays a role.* Civil Eats. https://civileats.com/2020/05/05/people-of-color-are-at-greater-risk-of-covid-19-systemic-racism-in-the-food-system-plays-a-role/

Parish, H. (2020). The absence of presence and the presence of absence: Social distancing, sacraments, and the virtual religious community during the COVID-19 pandemic. *Religions, 11*(6), 276.

Peacock, W. G., Van Zandt, S., Zhang, Y., & Highfield, W. E. (2014). Inequities in long-term housing recovery after disasters. *Journal of the American Planning Association, 80*(4), 356–371.

Pitsillides, S., & Wallace, J. (2021). *Physically distant but socially connected: Streaming funerals, memorials and ritual design during COVID-19* (pp. 60–76). https://doi.org/10.4324/9781003125990-4-6

Ramsetty, A., & Adams, C. (2020). Impact of the digital divide in the age of COVID-19. *Journal of the American Medical Informatics Association : JAMIA, 27*(7), 1147–1148. https://doi.org/10.1093/jamia/ocaa078

Rinde, M. (2020, July 7). Philadelphia opens spraygrounds, officials say they're safe for kids. *WHYY.* https://whyy.org/articles/spraygrounds-a-relatively-safe-way-to-cool-off-experts-say/

Roesch, E., Amin, A., Gupta, J., & Garcia-Moreno, C. (2020). Violence against women during covid-19 pandemic restrictions. *BMJ, 369.* https://doi.org/10.1136/bmj.m1712

Ruiz, N. G., Horowitz, J. M., & Tamir, C. (2020, July 1). Many black and Asian Americans say they have experienced discrimination amid the COVID-19 outbreak. *Pew Research Center's Social & Demographic Trends Project.* https://www.pewresearch.org/social-trends/2020/07/01/many-black-and-asian-americans-say-they-have-experienced-discrimination-amid-the-covid-19-outbreak/

Russo, M. (2021, August 2). *A cross-country comparison of contact-tracing apps during COVID-19.* CEPR. https://cepr.org/voxeu/columns/cross-country-comparison-contact-tracing-apps-during-covid-19

Sanderson, D. (2000). Cities, disasters and livelihoods. *Risk Management, 2*(4), 49–58.

Shutters, S. T. (2021). Modelling long-term COVID-19 impacts on the US workforce of 2029. *PLoS One, 16*(12), 1–17. a9h.

Su, Z., McDonnell, D., Roth, S., Li, Q., Šegalo, S., Shi, F., & Wagers, S. (2021). Mental health solutions for domestic violence victims amid COVID-19: A review of the literature. *Globalization & Health, 17*(1), 1–11. a9h.

Thomas, D. S., Phillips, B. D., Fothergill, A., & Blinn-Pike, L. (2009). *Social vulnerability to disasters*. CRC Press.

Toh, A., & Brown, D. (2020, June 4). *How digital contact tracing for COVID-19 could worsen inequality. Human Rights Watch*. https://www.hrw.org/news/2020/06/04/how-digital-contact-tracing-covid-19-could-worsen-inequality

van Dijk, J. A. G. M. (2006). Digital divide research, achievements and shortcomings. *Poetics, 34*(4–5), 221–235. https://doi.org/10.1016/j.poetic.2006.05.004

Van Orden, K. A., Bower, E., Beckler, T., Rowe, J., & Gillespie, S. (2022). The use of robotic pets with older adults during the COVID-19 pandemic. *Clinical Gerontologist, 45*(1), 189–194. a9h.

Vasel, Kathryn (2021, June 23). How PepsiCo is Rethinging the Office: More remote work. No assigned desks. *CNN*. https://www.cnn.com/2021/06/23/success/pepsi-return-to-work-plans/index.html

Weise, K. (2021, April 29). Amazon's profit soars 220 percent as pandemic drives shopping online. *The New York Times*. https://www.nytimes.com/2021/04/29/technology/amazons-profits-triple.html

Wells, J. (2020, May 27). *Coronavirus pandemic forces the funeral industry online*. CNBC. https://www.cnbc.com/2020/05/27/coronavirus-pandemic-forces-the-funeral-industry-online.html

Wiederhold, B. K. (2020). Turning to faith and technology during the coronavirus disease 2019 crisis. *Cyberpsychology, Behavior, and Social Networking, 23*(8), 503–504. https://doi.org/10.1089/cyber.2020.29191.bkw

Wienrich, C., Fries, L., & Latoschik, M. E. (2022). Remote at court. In G. Salvendy & J. Wei (Eds.), *Design, operation and evaluation of mobile communications* (pp. 82–106). Springer International Publishing. https://doi.org/10.1007/978-3-031-05014-5_8

Wisner, B. B., & Cannon, P. (2004). *At risk: Natural hazards, people's vulnerability and disasters*. Routledge.

Yang, C.-C., Tsai, J.-Y., & Pan, S. (2020). Discrimination and well-being among Asians/Asian Americans during COVID-19: The role of social media. *Cyberpsychology, Behavior and Social Networking, 23*(12), 865–870. https://doi.org/10.1089/cyber.2020.0394

Index

Pages in *italics* refer to figures and pages in **bold** refer to tables.